J. Thomas Lambrecht

3-D Modeling Technology
in Oral and Maxillofacial Surgery

3-D Modeling Technology in Oral and Maxillofacial Surgery

J. Thomas Lambrecht,
Prof. Dr. med. dent. Dr. med.

Chairman, Department of Oral Surgery,
-Radiology and -Medicine
University of Basel, Switzerland

quintessence
books

Quintessence Publishing Co, Inc
Chicago, Berlin, London, Tokyo, São Paulo,
Moscow, Prague, Sofia, and Warsaw

Library of Congress Cataloging-in-Publication Data

Lambrecht, J. Thomas (Jörg Thomas).
    3-D modeling technology in oral and maxillofacial surgery / J. Th. Lambrecht.
        p. cm.
        Includes bibliographical references.
        ISBN 0-86715-287-7
        1. Maxilla–Surgery–Simulation methods. 2. Face–Surgery
    –Simulation methods. 3. Mouth–Surgery–Simulation methods.
    4. Facial bones–Models. 5. Three–dimensional imaging in medicine.
    6. Moulage in medicine. 7. CAD/CAM systems. I. Title. II. Title:
    Three dimensional modeling technology in oral and maxillofacial surgery.
        [DNLM: 1. Mouth–surgery. 2. Surgery, Oral–methods. 3. Image
    Processing, Computer–Assisted–methods. 4. Models, Anatomic.
    WU 600 L226z 1995]
    RD526.L26   1995
    617.5'22059–dc20
    DNLM/DLC
    for Library of Congress   94-48366
                                                                          CIP

quintessence
books

© 1995 by Quintessence Publishing Co, Inc Carol Stream, Illinois,
All rights reserved.

Published by Quintessence Publishing Co, Inc
551 North Kimberly Drive 60188

Lithography: Color Line, Verona
Composition, Printing and Binding: Bosch-Druck, Landshut

Printed in Germany

ISBN 0-86715-287-7

Contents

3. Case Studies

Foreword

It is an honor to be invited to write the introduction for a new book; it is a privilege to do so for a respected colleague who happens also to be a friend. Common interest in the application of digital imaging and computer graphics to the analysis and reconstruction for acquired and congenital craniomaxillofacial deformities initiated our acquaintance. Over the years, we have come to know each other not just as investigators and health-care providers but also as individuals. Lest the reader of this foreword assume that friendship blinds critical review, let us say that familiarity provides a perspective for assessment that would be absent in the sterile analysis of a publication isolated from the vitality of its author.

The technological revolution, beginning in the nineteenth century, affected medicine and dentistry early with the development of radiography. The use of x-rays to produce images extended the physician and surgeon's indirect assessment of the living body beyond the examiner's personal senses of sight, hearing, touch, smell, and taste. The synchronous blossoming of surgery as an elective, rather than an emergency, activity and the subsequent development of antibiotics through the current century increased the need for accurate subsurface anatomic information. In addition to visualization of bones, internal cavities, and organs, radiography produced

documentation that could be analyzed by multiple observers without the presence of the patient. Such images allowed objective comparisons of findings in one individual over time or of multiple individuals with similar pathologic conditions.

At first, radiography was restricted to a few specialized facilities that had the technology. X-ray machines soon became commercial products that proliferated in hospitals and practitioners' offices alike. While interpretation of the images produced by radiography was initially performed by the examiner, over the last half century a specialized group of professionals, i.e., radiologists, evolved with expertise in interpretation of shadowy roentgenographic images. Medical practitioners have become increasingly dependent, to a much greater degree than practitioners in the dental medical field, on radiologists.

The benefit to patients from radiology is well established. Now, a century after Roentgen's initial x-ray image, new technologies of imaging living bodies have become available: ultrasonography, nuclear medicine, computerized tomographic (CT) scanning, magnetic resonance imaging (MRI), and positron emission tomography (PET).

Reflecting the absence of radiation in many of these technologies, the discipline has been renamed "diagnostic medical imaging" in many health-care facilities. Coincident with the development of imaging without the use of ionizing radiation, there has been continuing improvement in the anatomic fidelity of the images produced.

Digital imaging methods for the acquisition and processing of anatomic data is rapidly approaching the quality and detail previously available only through photography of autopsy or surgical specimens. Electronic in vivo "dissection" has become a reality and reference electronic atlases are being produced. Some investigators and clinicians, however, are more interested in spatial anatomic details and their quantitation than diagnosis per se. These professionals tend not to be radiologists. They adapted conventional roentgenography to the study of skulls through cephalometry in the first quarter of this century, and have led the consumer demand for new methods of display of contemporary computer-assisted imaging.

The data acquired by digital imaging and computer graphics technology can be expressed in a number of ways that have proven useful to students of anatomy and health-care providers alike. Initially the data were displayed as simple transaxial "slices." The ability to reformat collections of slice data into planes orthogonal to that of the data acquisition process improved the utility of the data and often obviated the need for additional radiation dose and/or scanning procedures. While the slice format remains the preferred mode of presentation for most radiologists, for the diagnostic interpreters of such information, the discordance of slice format with the reality of the examination room or the operative suite limits its utility in planning and delivering therapy. Health-care providers deal with patients as surfaces and volumes, and not as slices, a format limited to patholo-

gists. The reformation of digital imaging data into three-dimensional surface or volume images, initially osseous and then soft tissue as well, expanded the utility of the data to quantitative anatomic evaluation for dysmorphology study, surgical planning, outcome evaluation, and education. The appeal of such surface images resides in the universal iconography, for both medical and lay persons alike, of the human skull: a familiar icon. In less than a decade, three-dimensional surface reformations from CT scans have matured from a novelty of the early 1980s into an essential element of craniofacial assessment and communication in the 1990s.

The interaction and manipulation of these three-dimensional images were limited by their availability as either soft-copy cathode-ray tube (CRT) images or static hard-copy on transparent film. While 3-D workstations became available synchronously with the development of surface imaging technology, the cost of such workstations was initially prohibitive for most potential end-users. Dramatic improvements in desktop computing power at relatively low cost and the development of commercially available medical 3-D imaging software have made 3-D workstations affordable for most practical applications. Interrogation of the 3-D imaging database using such workstations allows registration of serial images, thereby obviating the problem of random head positioning during CT or MRI data acquisition, superimposition of selected hard and soft tissues, interactive surgical simulation, and evaluation of change over time due to growth, aging, or intervention.

Computer imaging of the skeleton was quickly adapted for the fabrication of custom implants to replace damaged or missing portions. While such custom pros-

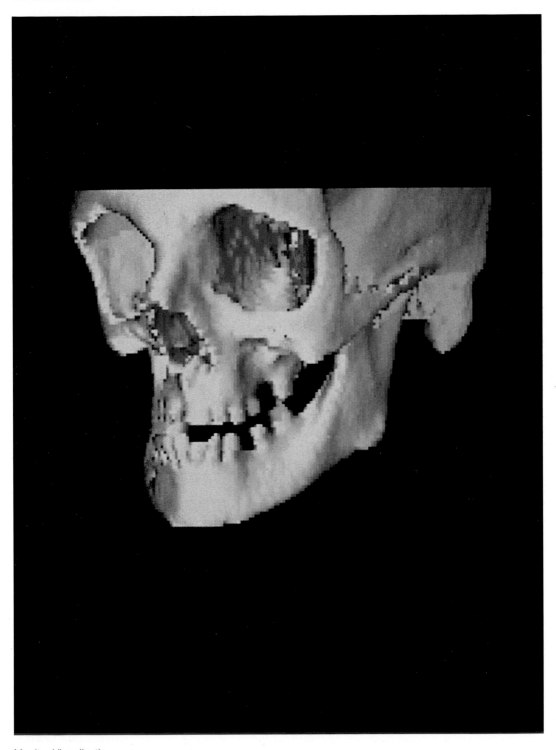

Monitor Visualisation

theses were initially designed on workstations and then milled using computer-aided design and manufacturing (CAD/CAM) technology from discrete manufacturing, fabrication of anatomical replicas soon followed. Instead of relying on a cadaveric museum specimen or an artist's sculpted body part, clinicians can examine these facsimiles for their geometric qualities and manipulate and modify a realistic facsimile, unique to the individual who will be treated, of the anatomic part in question.

The fabrication of space-filling, fully three-dimensional anatomic replicas has become an important alternative presentation of the 3-D data base acquired by CT or MR scanning. Such facsimiles are immediately attractive to anatomists and health-care providers unfamiliar with interactive computer-graphics technology since these models resemble the museum specimens of the anatomy laboratory. Although the production of such facsimiles requires sophisticated computer technology, utilization of the facsimiles is possible far from the computer hardware itself and by computer illiterati. The replicas can be examined manually, cut with surgical tools to practice known operations or to simulate novel ones, and used to fabricate custom implants or prebend internal fixation devices. As with all technology, there are limitations. Model surgery is, necessarily, a destructive process, and a trial of alternative operations requires a new facsimile for each attempt. Furthermore, facsimile fabrication at this time involves both significant time and expense.

Beyond the issue of whether or not to fabricate space-filling, life-sized facsimiles is the question of which technology and which materials are best for fabrication. Initially these facsimiles were fabricated using industrial, numerically controlled multiaxis milling machines. Construction of similar machine tools dedicated to the needs of body part fabrication soon developed. While facsimiles so produced provide excellent single-surface, whether exocranial or endocranial, replication, the ability to produce a skull facsimile with anatomic fidelity of both internal as well as external surfaces is limited with milling machines. Stereolithography, a technology introduced in the 1980s, has excellent capability to produce very complex objects. However, the prolonged manufacturing time and marked expense of this fabrication process are serious impediments to its wide application. Whether facsimile milling from solid blocks or stereolithographic photopolymerization of liquids will dominate and endure, or whether both will continue to be used for specific applications, is yet to be determined.

Beyond the questions of technical feasibility and clinical utility, the technologies of image acquisition and display must be considered in the context of health-care in general. Computer-assisted medical imaging is not inexpensive. Increasing alarm in most developed countries over seemingly uncontrollable health-care costs compels one to question the utility of such technology. This work of Lambrecht joins that of others in documenting the clinical application of that technology. Accurate preoperative skull facsimile surgery decreases intraoperative time by providing the surgeon with a quantitative skeletal surgical blueprint, eliminating unanticipated spatial conflicts among mobilized bones, and transferring rigid fixation plate coaptation from the intraoperative to preoperative period. Decreased operative time reduces costs directly in a health-care system where such charges are temporally related

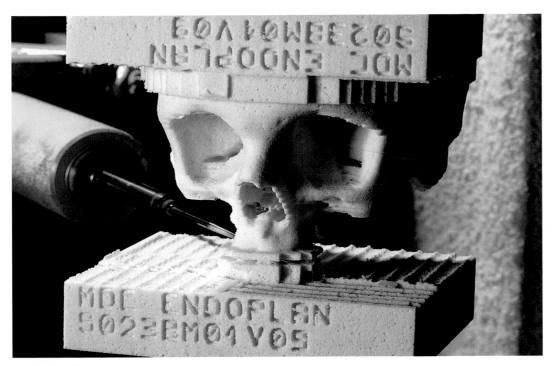

Model Fabrication

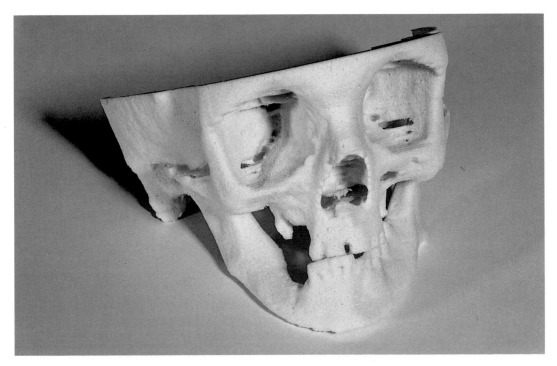

Individual 3-D Model

(the USA) and indirectly by decreasing operative complications, which have been directly related to length of operative time. Less easily quantitated but significant is an improved ability to train new surgeons through realistic simulation rather than through human trial and error.

Dr. Lambrecht and coworkers in Kiel, Germany, were pioneers in this application. They demonstrated the feasibility of milling skull facsimiles and documented the clinical utility of such models in the presurgical preparation for management of dentoskeletal deformities. This text richly documents Dr. Lambrecht's broad experience in the field and confirms his position as one of the international leaders in the application of computer-assisted imaging to facsimile fabrication and utilization. Much as the industrial product designer eventually transforms the computer design to a spatial prototype, so is it probable that both the manipulation of computer images on a 3-D workstation and the fabrication of life-size facsimiles will continue to provide useful information to both investigative and clinical health-care professionals. These two methods of data display should not be considered in competition but as complementary, providing the end-user with the best possible access to the diagnostic imaging data.

The application of advanced computer graphics and image synthesis to diagnostic medical imaging has produced improved technology for anatomic investigation, surgical simulation, and postoperative follow-up. Increased anatomic comprehension and a quantitative, geometrically accurate capability have made this technology essential for the evaluation and management of both congenital and acquired craniofacial deformities. The continued development of image acquisition and display hardware and software should facilitate the utility of this technology and provide new, as yet unimagined, applications for health-care use. *3-D Modeling Technology in Oral and Maxillofacial Surgery* is an important way station along the path to that future.

Jeffrey L. Marsh, M.D.
Professor of Surgery
Division of Plastic and
Reconstructive Surgery
Washington University School of Medicine
St. Louis, Missouri

Michael W. Vannier, M.D.
Professor of Radiology
Mallinckrodt Institute of Radiology
Washington University School of Medicine
St. Louis, Missouri

Preface

The term *3-D* seems to have a magic touch nowadays. There is a significant difference between monitor visualization (CAD, computer-aided design) showing the third dimension perspectively and solid models filling out the third dimension in space (CAM, computer-aided manufacturing). The manufacture of individual models of patients' skeletal structures opens surgeons' horizons. The rapidly proceeding technological development is of determinating importance. Computer-aided surgery (CAS) will play an important role in the future. Only a team of interdisciplinary clinicians, scientists, technicians, and computer specialists can master the immeasurable amount of upcoming work.

Between 1985 and 1991, as a senior lecturer in the Department for Oral and Maxillofacial Surgery at the Christian Albrechts University hospital in Kiel, Germany, I had the good fortune to belong to such a team. The surgical procedures presented in this book were performed by the following:

Prof. Dr. Dr. F. Härle (Chairman); Prof. Dr. Dr. R. Ewers (today: Chairman, Department of Maxillofacial Surgery, University Hospital, Vienna, Austria); Prof. Dr. Dr. B. Hoffmeister (today: Chairman, Department of Maxillofacial Surgery, University Hospital Benjamin Franklin, Berlin, Germany); Prof. Dr. Dr. K. Wangerin (today: Co-Chairman, Department of Plastic Surgery, Marienhospital, Stuttgart, Germany); Priv. Doz. Dr. Dr. Th. Kreusch (today: Vice-chairman, Department of Maxillofacial Surgery, University Hospital, Kiel, Germany); and myself.

I thank my colleagues for their constructive support.

I would also like to thank:

Prof. Dr. F. Brix (today: Chairman, Department of Radiology, City Hospital, Kiel, Germany), without whom this project would never have had a start; Prof. Dr. H. Gremmel (Chairman Emeritus, Department of Radiology, University Hospital, Kiel, Germany); Priv. Doz. Dr. W. Zenker (Department of Traumatology, University Hospital in Kiel, Germany); Dipl. Math. D. Hebbinghaus, Dr. M. Behm, and Dr. J. Jalass, who were active team partners, offering ideas and putting in considerable effort; and H. Ihde, U. Kliegis, R. Schröder, W. Schwesig, and H. Weigel, who, with the companies they represent, supported the team; and Mrs. Dorothee Wurster, who typed the manuscript with cheerful diligence.

The purpose of this book is to address the opportunities offered by, and indications for 3-D modeling in oral and maxillofacial surgery. More specifically, the purpose is to reveal how 3-D technologies offer diagnostic and therapeutic advantages for patients in need of surgical treatment for neoplasms, malformations, dysgnathias, preprosthetic surgery, implants, and TMJ problems.

I am convinced that 3-D technology will be of ample importance in the surgical field. The technology's continuing development, now in its third generation, speaks for itself.

J. Thomas Lambrecht

1. Introduction

Oral and maxillofacial surgery must conform to high standards both for the rehabilitation of function and esthetics. This is especially true for surgical procedures involving large-scale remodeling, removal, or reconstruction of tissue. Accordingly, a thorough preoperative planning and preparation phase is imperative for surgical success.

Oral and maxillofacial surgery has long needed a methodology for accurate definition of the third dimension. The introduction of computer-aided radiotomography in the 1970s provided surgeons with multiple two-dimensional maps of information, which they themselves had to conceptualize into a third dimension. The later advent of computerized summation of these data made it possible to display a perspective view of the third dimension on a monitor.

Computerized tomography (CT) and, in parts, magnetic resonance tomography (MRT or MRI) data with the analytic refinement afforded by contour summation, visualization, model fabrication, and surgical planning allow for extensive methodical preoperative planning. Additionally, three-dimensional models of bony structures can now be made available for the planning and performance of surgical procedures on the skull. These models, which can be milled from a variety of materials, allow surgeons the opportunity to study the bony structures of a patient outside the body and to manipulate their shapes as required to achieve a desired result. Models permit the measurement of structures, the testing of osteotomic and resection techniques, and complete planning for almost all types of oral and maxillofacial surgery.

In addition to utility for preprosthetic and tumor surgery, three-dimensional modeling can assist in surgical correction of malocclusion and congenital deformities. In traumatology, however, its applications in primary care are limited due to time constraints. The future potential of modeling justifies continued expense of labor and costs in the manufacture of models, for three-dimensional surgical planning will shorten the time required for surgical procedures in oral and maxillofacial surgery.

General History of 3-D Technology

Until the early 1970s, surgeons depended mainly on diagnostic radiography, either in the form of summation radiographs or tomographs that were produced in two different planes. Being only two-dimensional, the images produced with these techniques fell short of a true spatial representation of the surgical space. The introduction and continued development of computer-aided radiotomography (Hounsfield 1973, Glenn et al. 1975) led to a rapid increase of information for various planes. Conceptualization of the third dimension, however, remained a serious problem. Pape et al. (1977) developed a device for measuring the symmetry of the center portion of the human face: the data were plotted on two-dimensional profile curves by means of an automatic plotter. Fritzemeier (1981) measured the facial relief optically with a projected grid in order to document the development of the initial status and changes of the facial contours. Kawano (1987) proposed the use of moire topography for three-dimensional facial morphometry, using photographs of the patient taken from different directions as a baseline. Kobayashi et al. (1990) developed a similar system for a three-dimensional analysis of the facial morphology before and after orthognathic surgery.

More recent developments of this methodology are reported by Meinzer et al. (1991) and Vannier et al. (1991). Speculand et al. (1984) used a "halo-caliper" to facilitate precise three-dimensional positioning of the segments during surgery. In traumatology, Hoffmeister et al. (1983) sought to determine the third dimension of mandibular osteosynthesis based on studies of cadavers.

The need for a representation or reconstruction of the third dimension had long been recognized in other fields. Mittermayer and Niederdellmann (1979), Kanz et al. (1980), and Baumann et al. (1990) studied the feasibility of using a sequence of histologic sections to produce true three-dimensional replicas of internal body structures. Scharfetter et al. (1986) reconstructed a juvenile ossifying fibroma with cardboard and resin models to determine, in addition to the histologic status, the growth

pattern and the biologic behavior of the tumor. In the field of dento-maxillofacial radiology, Lambrecht (1984) determined the third dimension of section contour and depth of panoramic radiographic apparatuses.

Early detection of tissue and organ diseases also required new techniques to facilitate precise diagnosis even in the initial stages of disease. Such techniques became feasible as imaging devices grew more sensitive. With CT, ultrasound echography, and MRT, a variety of imaging techniques capable of furnishing the quantitative data needed for diagnosis were developed. The desire to obtain a three-dimensional view of anatomic structures with the help of these technologies required that precise data on the surface relevant to the object to be imaged be made available. This information, for example, could be found in a sequence of CT scans; however, the information was distributed over a multitude of slices. With the help of enhanced electronic image interpretation, Liu (1977), Artzy (1979), and later Steinhäuser et al. (1987) succeeded in filtering out data specific to the desired surface and in displaying a three-dimensional perspective view of an object on a monitor. Visual imaging methods were further refined by Hemmy et al. (1983), and Vannier et al. (1984). Coded gray-tone imaging was improved by Chen et al. (1985), Gillespie and Isherwood (1986) and Gillespie et al. (1987). Cutting et al. (1986) took this work one step further with a report on experiences with surgical planning aided by computer images. Although three-dimensional (3-D) models were mentioned, their practical application was limited by technical problems.

It became evident that spatial conditions could be truly understood only with a three-dimensional model. Brix et al. (1985) intro-

16

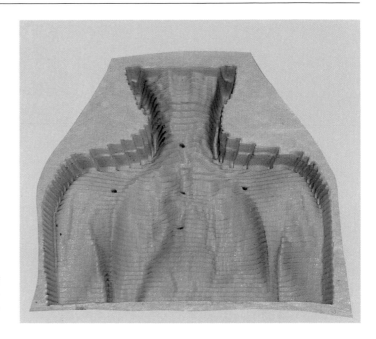

Fig. 1 Negative mold (Styrodur) of neck and thorax as used in radiotherapy for compensation techniques.

duced a process for controlling a milling machine (used in model fabrication), which permitted three-dimensional shaping of stock styrofoam pieces. Such models were fabricated as negative molds and used in radiotherapy for compensation techniques (Fig. 1). The first positive molds were milled following monitor visualization (Fig. 2) and were shaped by using a heated wire loop (Fig. 3). The results were not promising (Fig. 4).

The development of a new multiple axis milling machine and the application of an improved computer control program (Kliegis et al. 1988) made it possible to fabricate complete individual anatomic models, such as tubular bones of patients, entirely from one piece of stock material (Figs. 5 and 6).

Brix and Lambrecht (1987) first reported the fabrication of individual skull models based on CT data. With these develop-

ments, 3-D models of bone structures became available to the surgeon.

Visualization

Computer-generated perspective views can offer the surgeon an approximate spatial visualization of the third dimension of skeletal structures (Marsh and Vannier 1983a and b, Hemmy et al. 1983, Pate et al. 1986, Witte et al. 1986, DeMarino et al. 1986, Pate et al. 1987, Ernsting et al. 1987, Gillespie 1988, Schellhas et al. 1988, White 1988, Zinreich et al. 1988, Engelmann et al. 1989, Lang et al. 1989, Zonneveld et al. 1989, Fishman et al. 1990, Hildeboldt et al. 1990, Vannier 1991, Wallin 1991, Mutoh et al. 1991, Udupa and Odhner 1991).

Especially in case of complex fractures of the facial portion of the skull, this method

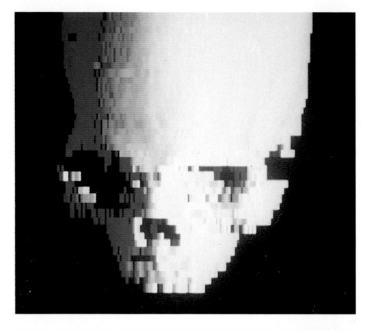

Fig. 2 Early version of 3-D perspective monitor visualization of a human skull using interpreted CT scan data.

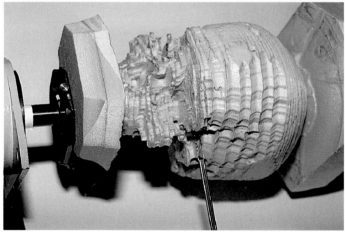

Fig. 3 Milling of a 3-D skull model using an electrically heated wire loop.

can be a significant aid in planning reconstructive therapy (Grodd et al. 1987). Hirschfelder et al. (1989) used a computer monitor to reconstruct the three-dimensional surfaces of bony structures in regions that prohibit radiographic access. Certain congenital asymmetries, such as hemifacial microsomia or other craniofacial anomalies are standard indications for three-dimensional processing using CT data (Ono et al. 1989, Matsuno et al. 1990, Whyte et al. 1990, Strong et al. 1990.

In 1985, Arridge et al. discussed the possibility of using computer aided design (CAD) as a tool for planning and simulation in reconstructive facial surgery. This me-

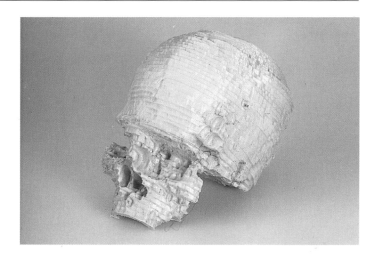

Fig. 4 Result of first attempt at producing a 3-D skull model (prototype).

thod was based on data acquisition using a laser in combination with a TV camera. Bhatia and Sowray (1984) and Walters and Walters (1986) used two-dimensional planning programs for orthognathic surgery. Hunt and Rudge (1984) combined such a program with the superimposition of photographs. Haskell et al. (1986) "modeled" on the screen interpreting two-dimensional data. Imhof (1989) proposed a temporary conversion to "wireframe" images for schematic visualization and processing. According to Katagiri et al. (1987), CT offered the opportunity to analyze the three-dimensional structure via serial scans in the diagnosis of alveolar bone defects as well as with implants (Schwarz et al. 1987a and b).

In the absence of ancillary devices, conversion of two-dimensional information to the third dimension was consigned to, and possibly constricted by, individual conceptual ability processes.

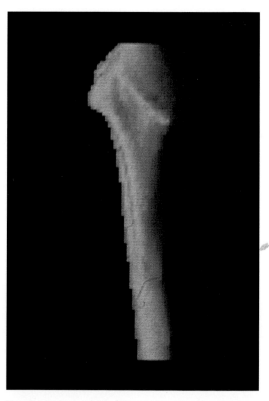

Fig. 5 Monitor visualization of a proximal humerus.

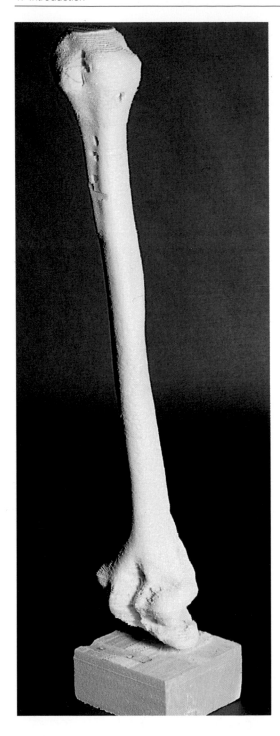

Fig. 6 Model of a human humerus milled from Styrodur.

With all these techniques, the surgeon was relegated to the passive role of an observer limited by his/her conceptual ability. Only through the purely visual image on the computer screen could he/she obtain an impression of the conditions at the site of surgery.

The most recent developments, such as stereotactic surgery controlled by CT for the diagnosis and treatment of neurosurgical diseases (Schachenwald et al. 1990), make use of three-dimensional technology in the form of computer-aided surgery (CAS). They represent an attempt to make the known three-dimensional data available to the surgeon for his/her use during an actual procedure (Adams et al. 1990).

Rapid advances in chip technology have made it possible to implement computer systems capable of processing highly differentiated problems within the CAD three-dimensional system while using only a minimum of memory (Pomaska 1987, Seldon 1991).

Multidimensional data information was recently specified and standardized through the American College of Radiology (Udupa et al. 1992).

Jalass (1992) visualized data from MRT, and Sohn et al. (1989) reported on the potential applicability of three-dimensional ultrasound images. Indeed, without exception, all two-dimensional data bases are viable sources for developing a visual representation of the third dimension in perspective.

Model Construction

The physical reproduction of structures visualized on a monitor was pursued independently by researchers in Germany (Brix et al. 1985, Brix and Lambrecht 1987,

Kliegis et al. 1988, Kliegis et al. 1990) and in the United States (Woolson et al. 1986, Pate et al. 1986), all started with the same basic idea: to produce three-dimensional models replicating the body structures of individual patients.

While German researchers focused on a direct milling process from the start (Brix 1981) to meet the needs of radiation therapy, American researchers (Donlon et al. 1988, Catone 1988, Guyuron and Ross 1989) pursued the concept of a two-stage model fabrication. In this process, a three-axis milling machine was used to mill two negative halfshellsed made of wax, which, when joined, formed a hollow casting mold. In a second step this mold was filled with a liquid resin. After curing, the wax was removed to reveal the finished resin model. A comparison of the two processes shows that direct milling wastes more high-quality model material. To date, no studies of comparative accuracy have been performed.

In 1985, Mildenstein et al. and Giebel et al. introduced a third process for the fabrication of models. CT data were fed into a computer-controlled laser cutter, which produced a series of slices. The slices were then glued together and the resulting steps smoothed mechanically. No information on the thickness of the slices was provided and it was not made clear whether the mechanical smoothing process was pre-programmed by interpolation.

Other methods include one propagated by Aldinger (Aldinger et al. 1984, Aldinger and Weigert 1991), which focuses on manufacturing hip endoprostheses. A further development of laser technology is stereolithography, in which liquid resin is polymerized layer-by-layer using UV laser. The polymerized layer is electromechanically dipped into a liquid monomer that, in turn, will be laser polymerized, as steered by a programmed computer. Repetitions of this process will eventually produce the model (Ghezal and Stucki 1992).

First reports explore the suitability of this method for surgical simulation and the manufacturing of implants (Palser et al. 1990, Mankovich et al. 1990, Klein et al. 1992, Stoker et al. 1992, Schmitz and Erbe 1992).

Limitations and Potential Applications

Three-dimensional model fabrication continues to require high-volume data processing and extensive computation. In addition, the milling process requires constant supervision in its initial stages. Because the labor-intensive nature of the process does not yet permit routine application in acute therapeutic surgical procedures, the benefits of three-dimensional model fabrication are compromised by the expense of equipment and its maintenance. Broader, interdisciplinary utilization would make the technique more cost-effective.

Another limiting factor is the system's inability to produce satisfactory soft tissue analyses, or to allow reliable prognoses in this respect. Computerized two-dimensional processes for soft tissue analysis are already available (Hing 1989). However, the three-dimensional perspective, which, for example, is crucial for discussing likely outcomes of surgery with a patient, is lacking. Although the skeleton can be modeled well, and the symmetry of skeletal parts can usually be achieved in model surgery, there is no guarantee that soft tissue segments will yield comparable symmetry. In other words, 3-D technology falls short of being entirely satisfactory for approximation of esthetic outcomes.

21

Finally, the radiation exposure of a CT scan is a further limiting factor in the decision to construct and use a 3-D model. In our experience CT scans for surgical planning in the central facial and mandibular region should exclude the radiation-sensitive orbital region, with the first section being taken no higher than the orbital floor.

This, however, only holds true for sagittal problems. Transverse asymmetries and craniofacial anomalies always require replicas of the entire skeletal structure of the head, to determine the correct sagittal, transverse and horizontal planes.

MRT data are of somewhat limited value for the contouring of skeletal structures (Jalass 1992). The approximate contouring of adjacent soft tissue and newly developed subtraction methods are expected to be improved in the future. The use of MRT data as basic information will also have an influence on the utility of model fabrication in related disciplines. It is already possible to produce three-dimensional models of the brain, liver, or heart (Jalass 1992).

In orthopedic traumatologic surgery, Zenker et al. (1990a and b) were able to reclassify the fractures of the calcaneus on the basis of model fabrication. This opens up entirely new perspectives for the solution of orthopedic problems, such as those involved in fabrication of custom endoprostheses for the hip joint.

Volumetric quantifications of intracranial and ventricular volumes for follow-up after craniofacial surgery were performed in 1987 by Dufresne et al. In 1990, Höhne et al. and Tiede et al. gave access to new dimensions with a special algorithm: slice by slice, internal body structures could be subtracted or added. With MRT data acquisition, examinations of this type are possible at any time and without exposure to radiation.

Combining MRT data with positron emission tomography (PET) technology, Hu et al. (1990) were able to represent metabolic processes three-dimensionally in terms of volume and extent, and the work of Kikinis et al. (1990) was aimed in the same direction. Further applications are suggested for the fields of neuroradiology (Zinreich et al. 1990) and radiation therapy (Schlegel 1990).

As to the precision of the models, Lill et al. (1991) and Solar et al. (1992) showed that polyurethane with an average accuracy of 1.6 mm is superior to Styrodur with an average accuracy of 2.1 mm. The total deviation of the polyurethane model from the dimensions of the original skull was 1.8% (Solar et al. 1992).

The conversion of three-dimensional data remains somewhat unsatisfactory in the occlusal area. Currently, the plaster models obtained with the help of impression materials are inserted in the styrofoam models with a SAM facebow. In the field of material science, Kinney et al. (1988) have developed a three-dimensional CT process aiming for a resolution of one micrometer. In this respect, computer-aided technologies (Stoll and Stachniss 1990) will offer as yet unimaginable accuracy in the future. Use of the reflex microscope or the reflex metrograph, an optical printer (Speculand et al. 1988a and b), may also hold promise.

Düchting (1988) is pursuing the development of prognostic models for the three-dimensional growth of tumors. His ultimate goal is to design optimal therapy with the help of computer experimentation. Attempts are being made to bring the model shape closer to reality with CT images. Three-dimensional processing on the cellular scale is being considered by Stevens et al. (1990).

The custom fabrication of individual skull models based on CT data and video visualization may also serve as a tool for successful skull identification in forensic medicine. For now, this method represents the culmination of a development driven by technological progress. In 1959, Grüner and Reinhard published a photographic method; Helmer and Grüner (1977) incorporated video technology in the superprojection technique; and barely a decade later, Pesce Delfino et al. (1986) reported their results using computer-aided superimposition techniques.

Lewin et al. (1990) also used three dimensional reconstructions when examining Egyptian mummies and emphasized, just as Hildeboldt et al. (1990), the value of this noninvasive new method in anthropology. Kreiborg et al. (1993) found very satisfactory results in the comparative three-dimensional analysis of the calvaria and cranial base in patients with Apert's syndrome and Crouzon's disease.

Applications in Oral and Maxillofacial Surgery

Currently, it is possible to mill models from a wide variety of materials, such as resin (Brix and Lambrecht 1987, Brix et al. 1988, Lambrecht et al. 1989, Zenker et al. 1990) or metal (Niederdellmann et al. 1988).

Actual fabrication of facsimile models was performed in our center with a five-axis milling machine. This enabled a direct manufacture of models out of any suitable material (Kliegis et al. 1988). This also gives us the capability to test new and higher-quality model materials in the future. Custom-milled implants will be made from allotropic biomaterials (Schmitz et al. 1990).

Results that are more accurate than those described by Waite and Matukas (1986) can be expected for the planning and the outcome of surgical procedures.

Three-dimensional models offer unique opportunities to study and manipulate bony structures outside the body (Zinreich et al. 1988). The complete reproduction of the spatial conditions inherent to the technique also offers the opportunity to take measurements of the mandibular model (Kursunoglu et al. 1986), to custom fit prostheses and maxillary or mandibular implants (Rhodes et al. 1987, Ono et al. 1993, Ross et al. 1993), and to test planned osteotomic and resection procedures (Guyuron and Ross 1989). For the reconstruction of bony defects, the necessary amount of graft material can be determined prior to surgery using three-dimensional modeling (Toth et al. 1988).

Planning of certain procedures in preprosthetic surgery (Kreusch and Lambrecht 1992) is possible with the aid of individual model fabrication as is presurgical preparation in primary reconstructions after tumor surgery (Hoffmeister and Lambrecht 1990). Surgical simulation in functional skeletal facial surgery (Lambrecht and Brix 1990a) and in orthognathic surgery (Lambrecht and Brix 1989 and 1990b) or craniofacial surgery (Lambrecht and Brix 1990c, Zonneveld and Van der Dussen 1992, Kärcher 1992, Yab et al. 1993) has been demonstrated.

The planning of surgical procedures with the help of a model has a keen advantage in that the surgical conditions can be simulated in an environment that closely reproduces the actual conditions. Thus, surgical strategy can be developed based on a clear view of the surgical site. This helps reduce the time needed to complete the actual procedure and, consequently, the

23

period of anesthetization, and it lowers the patient's risk of infection (Lambrecht and Brix 1989). Additionally, the model is very helpful in explaining the planned surgical procedure to the patient.

Three-dimensional models are ideally suited for a hands-on demonstration of surgical procedures (Frohberg and Haase 1993) in basic and advanced training of surgical personnel (Ellis 1990), and for testing planned osseous incisions.

The useful features of three-dimensional models based on CT and MRT data make them eminently suitable for application in almost all types of oral and maxillofacial surgery. In addition to preprosthetic and cancer surgery, this includes the therapy of maxillomandibular deformities and the surgical correction of malocclusion.

The enormous potential and advantages of the technology justify the current labor-intensive and cost-intensive fabrication of models. Finally, continued advances in the development of parallel (relational) computation (transputer) and faster programs (Ono et al. 1992, Kageyama et al. 1992, Kimura and Koga 1993) will further reduce the time (and the cost) required for model fabrication.

2. The 3-D Modeling Process

Computerized Tomography

To make the modeling process clear, we provide the following explication of what we've done:

The starting point for model fabrication is a series of CT scan sections of the patient. This series of images is then transferred into the computer (*see* Transfer of CT Images and Transfer of MRT Images). While reviewing the slice images, the contours of relevant structures are determined (*see* Contour Determination). From these contour data, the computer generates the surface data required for milling the model surfaces (*see* Calculation of Milling Tracks). A summation of the contours is displayed on a monitor, as well as a three-dimensional perspective view, in color, of the later model (*see* Visualization). The finished models (*see* Model Fabrication) are then used for further planning of the anticipated surgical procedure. The entire process is shown schematically in Fig. 7.

CT Images

Before a model can be fabricated, the respective bone structure (or part thereof) must be covered completely by a sequence of CT scans. We initially used a computerized tomograph made by the Picker company (Synerview 600) with a detector ring driven by a linear motor, and a 32-bit INTERDATA computer, model 7/32.

The content of the images showed a direct relation to the patient's position inside the computer tomograph. The patient's head in an overextended position gave coronal slice images. On the resulting model, the medioventral and dorsal surfaces showed a loss of surface information (Fig. 8).

With axial alignment of the patient, the scan sections were made parallel to the occlusal plane of the patient's teeth. (Fig. 9). The circumference of the mandible is shown in each slice. When fabricating a model of the central portion of the face, it is not always necessary to scan the radiation-sensitive orbital area.

It is imperative during the scanning process that the head of the patient be kept immobile in the initial rest position. Even slight turning or nodding motions of the head interfere with the proper sequence of the scans. In the resulting model, such undesirable artifacts of motion are visible as sharp-edged steps in the surface relief.

To prevent unintentional changes of the head position, a fully contoured head rest, a strap passing over the forehead (Fig. 10), or a custom-molded face mask may prove helpful. With children up to the age of five

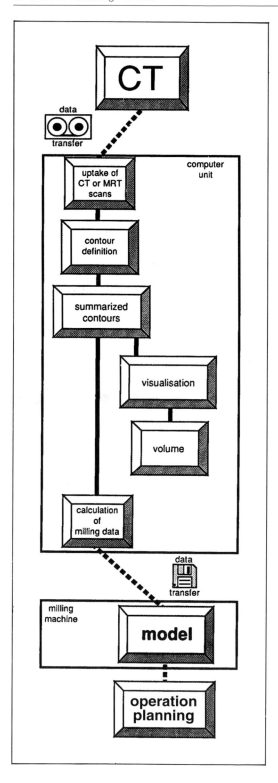

years, CT scans may be performed using intubation anesthesia.

To facilitate a clear distinction between the maxillary and mandibular arches for the determination of the slice contours, we used a custom-made, radiolucent occlusal splint. Dental restorations (fillings), fixed partial dentures, and orthodontic appliances caused centrifugal radiating artifacts in individual scans, obscuring structures that were of interest and inhibiting the definition of essential contours. For this reason, whenever feasible all artifact-producing structures were removed during patient preparation for the CT scan.

The number of section images per scan was determined by the skull size, the originally selected thickness of the individual sections, and the distance of the sections from each other.

Model quality can be improved with the following measures:

- A higher matrix (pixel resolution of the scan image)
- A larger number of slices
- A reduced slice thickness (2 mm)
- Secure positioning of the patient, and
- A short exposure time

Depending on the number of sections to be scanned, patients may have spent between 60 and 75 minutes in the computerized tomograph. In each section, decreases in radiation strength were recorded; using these data, the computer reconstructed mathematically a density distribution of each patient cross-section. A certain density value was assigned to each ab-

Fig. 7 Schematic view of process steps.

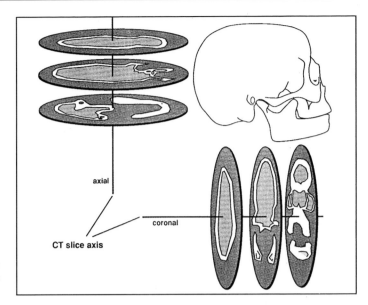

Fig. 8 Series of coronal and axial scans with related information content.

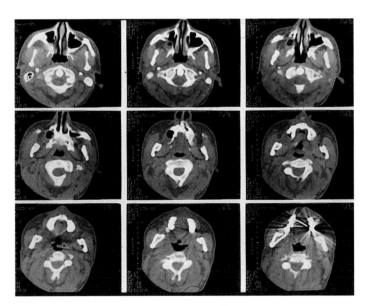

Fig. 9 Series of axial CT scans of the maxilla and the mandible, with the orbital area excluded.

sorption coefficient. The Hounsfield Density Scale (Gmelin 1987) ranges from −1000 to +1000 (−1000 = density of air / ±0 = density of water / 0 to 1000 = density > water). Like a mosaic, each slice consisted of 65,536 (256 × 256) density pixels.

For further processing, the data were transferred to magnetic tape.

To keep track of the procedure, we designed a checklist that could be used for the CT data and for fabrication records for the three-dimensional models (Table 1).

Table 1. CT Data Checklist

Patient Data:

Last name & first name:	Number:
Date of birth:	Examination date:
Ward/Physician:	Examined organ:
Remarks:	ID-No.:

Scan Data:

Matrix size:	Number of sections:
Table feed rate (mm):	Section thickness (mm):
Orientation (head/feet):	Travel direction of couch:
Diameter (mm):	

3-D Models:

Name of Model:

Prefix:

Processed Sections:

Visualization:
– Number of interpolations:
– Length of sequence:
– Name of sequence (4 letters):
– Filtered:

Milling Process:
– Scale:
– Number of interpolations:
– Name of milling data file:

Pre-Milling:
– Tool No.:
– Number of tracks:

Finishing:
– Tool No.:
– Number of tracks:
– Feed offset:
– Interpolated slice thickness:

Block width (mm):

Block height (mm):

Block length (mm):

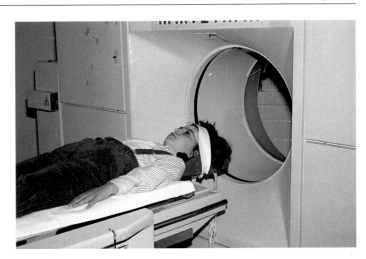

Fig. 10 Position and forehead strap for CT scans of an eight-year-old child.

Transfer of CT Images

We used an HP 9000 Series 300 computer as the central computer for model fabrication. It was based on a 16.7 MHz Motorola 68881 microprocessor, and was equipped with a Motorola 68020 math-coprocessor to support the extensive data-processing operations (Endoplan). The computer was configured with 3 MB of RAMS, a 30-MB hard disk, a 720-KB 3.5-inch disk drive, and an external tape drive with a tape capacity of 67 MB. An image storage and processing system (MEK-Imagine-MEDICAL) was integrated into the system. Additional peripherals included a monochrome 12-inch monitor, an RGB color monitor, a 107-key keyboard, an HP 46088A graphics tablet, and an HP 7475A plotter. The CT scan sequences of the patient were processed using proprietary software used in the ENDOPLAN 3-D program. The monitor displayed a touch-screen user interface with 14 starting fields (Fig. 11). Selection of COMTAPE activated the control program for the magnetic tape reader.

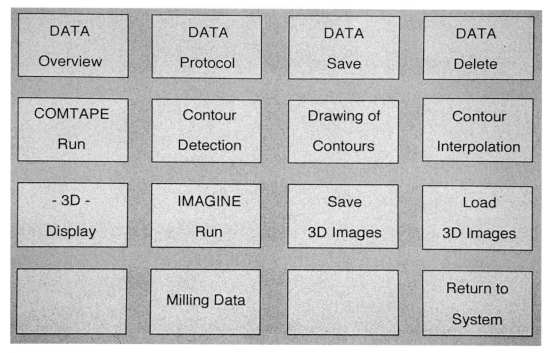

Fig. 11 User touch-screen monitor display.

The CT data of the patient could then be copied from the magnetic tape to the main computer.

For display on the monitor, an equivalent grayscale value had to be assigned to each density value. The computer supplied 252 grayscale values with linear distribution over the density interval of the Hounsfield scale.

To enhance the contrast, the software offered the option of assigning a disproportionately large number of grayscale values to sections of the Hounsfield scale. Thus, for density values between +80 and +400 (the so-called "special window"), grayscale images with higher differentiation could be displayed on the screen (Fig. 12).

Contour Determination

After transfer to the computer, the CT sections (slices) were reviewed individually on the screen, in strict ascending or descending sequence. To mark image sections and to control the processing, a screen cursor was used that was controlled by a digital pen on the graphics tablet (Fig. 13). Within the central square of the tablet, movements of the digital pen in the X and Y axis are reproduced as cursor movements on the screen.

The digital pen can also be used to enter figures via a numerical keypad. In addition, the following commands can be selected from the tablet: enlarge image segments (ZOOM), move slice images on the screen (MOVE SLICE), switch between preceding and following slices (SLICE FORW and SLICE BACKW), delete marked contours (DELETE CONT), or find contours in certain areas of the slice only (RESTRICT AREA).

The task in this case consisted of finding the bony margins of the mandible or of the skull in each of the sequence of slice images, and to mark the contours of the detected sections (Fig. 14). At the boundary between the bone and the surrounding soft tissue, a transition zone was found that was characterized by a rapid increase or decrease of density values (shown as different grayscales in Fig. 14). A Hounsfield density unit of +180 was measured at the level of the outer bone layer (compacta). The computer marked those areas of the image where the density reached or exceeded a value of +180. For this purpose, the computer systematically analyzed the density field of each slice image.

The starting point of the density analysis can be selected by the user to permit marking of selected portions of the image. All pixels located perpendicularly below the

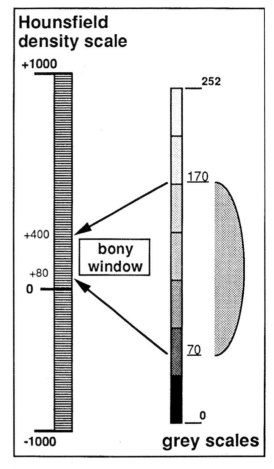

Fig. 12 Window for contrast enhancement.

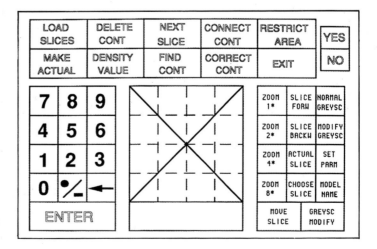

Fig. 13 Graphic tablet for operation with digital pen.

31

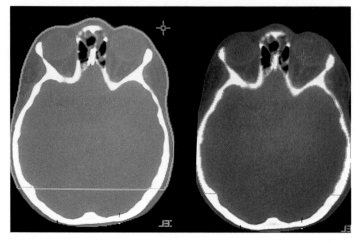

Fig. 14
Left: contour of soft tissue structures.
Bottom left: restriction of the contoured area (straight line).
Right: contour of skeletal structures (green line).

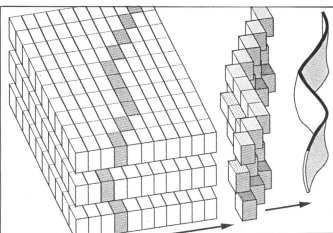

Fig. 15 Schematic of contour smoothing process.

cursor starting point were analyzed in succession for their density. The first pixel with a density exceeding the limit was the first point of the contour. The computer then analyzed the density of all adjacent pixels in clockwise fashion. Each additional pixel with a Hounsfield value exceeding the limit was added as another point of the contour to be determined. A contour was defined as an uninterrupted sequence of pixels. The program permitted a maximum of 3000 pixels per contour, and up to nine individu-

al contours per slice (so-called multiple contours).

The coarse and schematic curve of the contours (in a grid of 256 × 256 pixels) was smoothed by means of linear interpolation within each slice. In addition, the computer calculated a three-dimensionally curved surface, which enclosed all contours, smoothing them further (so-called "shell") (Chen et al. 1985). This "shell" provided for a smoother profile of the resulting model surface (Fig. 15). Following the image ana-

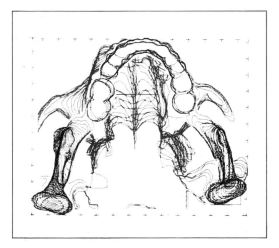

Fig. 16 Superimposed contour summation of maxilla (red) and mandible (black).

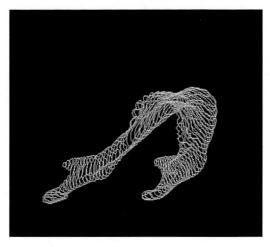

Fig. 17 Perspective view of the contour summation of a mandible.

lysis, the exact spatial coordinates of each contour were saved in a file (along with scale, position within the slice, and position of the slice).

Contour Summation

A three-dimensional model was generated by a three-dimensional assembly of all surface data, as determined by the analysis of the sequence of CT images. The surface in question could be reconstructed three-dimensionally from the sum of all contour pixels. First, all contours found during the analysis of the CT sequence were collected. Then, by using a plotter, all contours were superimposed on paper in original size (Fig. 16), with a metric coordinate system showing the sagittal and transverse extension.

In addition to the summary two-dimensional display of all contours, the following control function was available: by rotating

the perpendicular axis and by pulling apart the contours, a three-dimensional perspective view could be generated. This process step could be documented on the screen (Fig. 17) as well as on the HP plotter (Fig. 18).

Visualization

At this point, performing an additional visual check of the current state of the analysis offered certain advantages. It was possible to view the contoured skeletal structures of the patient's head perspectively in the form of a three-dimensional colored object on the monitor (Fig. 19). Errors that would have produced inaccuracies of the model surface became visible and could be corrected at this stage.

By adding an imaginary light source, the view of the object displayed on the screen could be enhanced. Different views of the object from different angles were com-

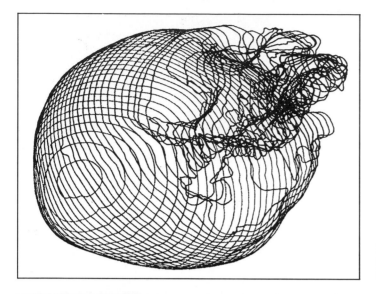

Fig. 18 Perspective view of the contour summation of a calotte printed by a plotter.

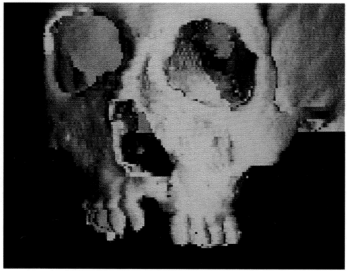

Fig. 19 Visualization of a patient's skull with alveolar process area after osteoplastic cleft surgery.

puted. When displayed in rapid sequence, a rotation of the object could be simulated. At this point it was possible to display the results of volumetric calculations as visualizations on the screen. Cavities, defects, or interponates to be fabricated are examples of volumetric calculations that might be converted to a three-dimensional perspective view.

34

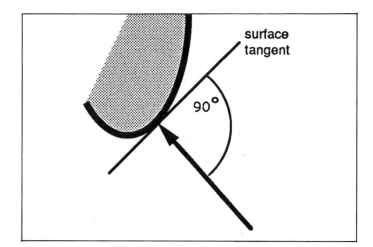

Fig. 20 Ideal angle of the milling tool relative to the surface being milled.

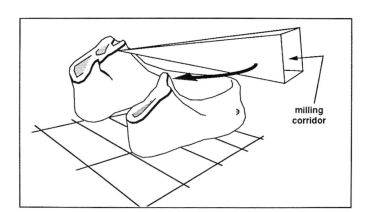

Fig. 21 Collision detection is calculated to protect model and milling tool.

Calculation of Milling Tracks

The computer calculated a sequence of control commands for the milling machine, based on all the previously determined surface points of the object to be fabricated and their spatial coordinates. The program offered the options of enlarging or reducing the overall size of the object to be milled, or to reverse its sides. Different shapes and sizes of cutting tools could also be applied. The actual milling process was designed so that the milling tool milled the contours sequentially slice after slice, following precisely the contours defined for each one. Our goal was to keep the milling tool perpendicular to the area of the model surface being milled (Fig. 20).

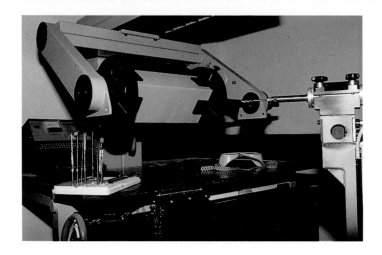

Fig. 22 CNC milling machine with clamped workpiece.

However, for complex surface structures like the mandible, it became necessary to deviate from this ideal cutting angle to avoid random collisions between the cutting tool and the model.

Through an ongoing simulation of the cutting process, the computer automatically checked whether the calculated milling tracks were correct (so-called collision detection) (Fig. 21). For this, the following information was needed:

a. The model surface at any point of the milling process
b. The angle between milling tool and model surface
c. The admissible angle between the milling tool and the perpendicular (milling corridor)
d. The diameter and the length of the milling tool.

The end result was a vector path that determined the coordinated movement of the milling tool in three dimensions. Also, a second vector path at a greater distance from the model surface was calculated to facilitate preshaping of the block of material. Finally, the computer displayed the required height, width, and length of the brick-shaped block of material from which the model was to be milled.

The computed milling control data were then transferred to 720-KB disks.

Model Fabrication

Milling Machine

The calculation of the milling data and the milling of the models were separate processes in terms of both time and space. By using a separate work space for the milling of the models, the noise level was reduced and a contamination of the computer area was avoided. The model was fabricated with a CNC milling machine (Fig. 22). The machine consisted of a table-like structure with a work surface made of hardwood. Above the work surface was the main arm, with a moving slide suspended from its underside. A workpiece basket capable of holding workpieces of different sizes by

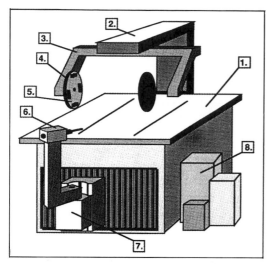

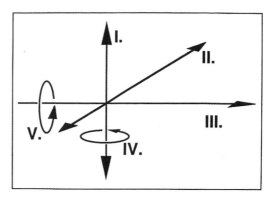

Fig. 24 Degrees of freedom (five) of the milling machine.

Fig. 23 Schematic view of the milling machine: 1 = work surface; 2 = main arm; 3 = slide; 4 = workpiece basket; 5 = workpiece; 6 = milling head; 7 = gear; 8 = spare workpieces.

means of interchangeable clamping plates was attached to the slide (Fig. 23). The milling head was moved by means of gears.

The system was designed for milling operations with five degrees of freedom (Fig. 24). In X and Y axes, the milling tool was capable of translational motions (I + II), and it rotated on a horizontal plane (IV). The workpiece basket moved linearly in the Z axis (III) and could be rotated 360 degrees with a defined passage through zero (V).

These motions were produced by five individual stepping motors that could be controlled independently and that were installed in a solid and vibration-resistant chassis. Motor control was provided by an HP Vectra microcomputer configured with a 3.5-inch disk drive and a 30-MB hard disk.

Model Materials

Suitable materials for model fabrication had to meet the following requirements:

1. Can be cut to the proper size for the intended purpose
2. Acceptable viscoelasticity
3. Stable shape and indefinite shelf life
4. Dense internal structure
5. Hardness comparable to bone
6. Heat and solvent resistant
7. Sterilizable
8. Color similar to bone.

The higher the volumetric weight (i.e., density) of the material,

- The more stable the milled model

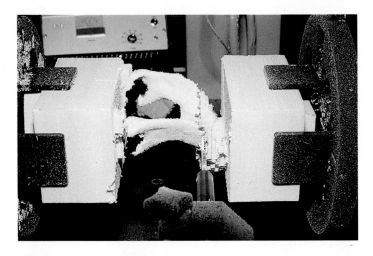

Fig. 25 Workpiece, Styrodur 5000 S, clamped in the workpiece basket during the milling process.

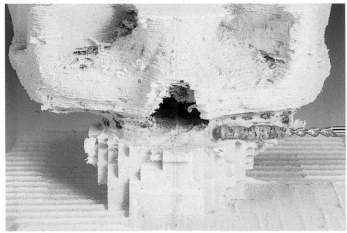

Fig. 26 Overheated styrofoam glued to the drill surface causes destruction of the model.

- The finer the structures that can be milled
- The more precise the model surface
- The less wear of the model surface
- The lower the risk of damage
- The slower the cutting speed during the milling process
- The sooner the cutting tool becomes dull
- The greater the danger of tool fracture.

Two foam materials had properties and processing characteristics that made them suitable for model fabrication: Styrodur and Polyurethane 200.

Styrodur 5000 S is a green, extruded, hard polystyrene foam material (Fig. 25). It was available in panels with a thickness of 8 cm, which can be glued together with two-component epoxy resin adhesive to

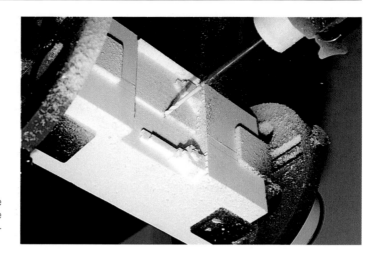

Fig. 27 Workpiece of Polyurethane 200, clamped in the workpiece basket at the start of the milling process.

form larger blocks. Due to its low volumetric weight, 50 kg/m^3, this material is also suitable for models of larger parts of the skeleton (eg, skull and pelvis).

A disadvantage of the material is a tendency to overheat occasionally, leading to model inaccuracies of varied extent (Fig. 26).

The nonporous closed-cell polyurethane foam used had a volumetric weight of 200 kg/m^3 (Fig. 27). It comes in panels with a thickness of 10 cm and is distinguished by its pale yellow color and great strength. A urethane foam, also yellow, served as an adhesive. With the help of a thixotropic agent, it was foamed to prevent the formation of crystalline structures.

Since the preparation of the workpieces always required gluing together at least two 10-cm panels, this type of adhesive layer, having the same physical properties as the workpiece material, did not interfere with milling.

When manipulated, the surface of the polyurethane foam was abraded, producing a sandy dust. We opted to seal the model surface with a transparent and heat-resistant spray enamel. The material can be sterilized by gas sterilization.

Milling Tools

Prior to precise milling of the surface details, the workpiece was coarsely milled to shape. This required selecting both coarse and fine milling tools from the range available. The specific selection depended on the model material. We used double-cutting carbide face cutters with clockwise rotation and counterclockwise chip-guiding grooves.

Polyurethane was premilled with special end-milling cutters with a shank diameter of 4 mm and a cutting edge width of 6 mm, and then finished with a cutting edge width of 1.5 mm. V$_2$A Hard Metal (VHM) copy milling tools proved to be suitable for milling the lighter styrofoam materials. With a tool length of 100 mm, the coarse cutters had a cutting edge width of 4 mm, and the finish cutters one of 1.2 mm.

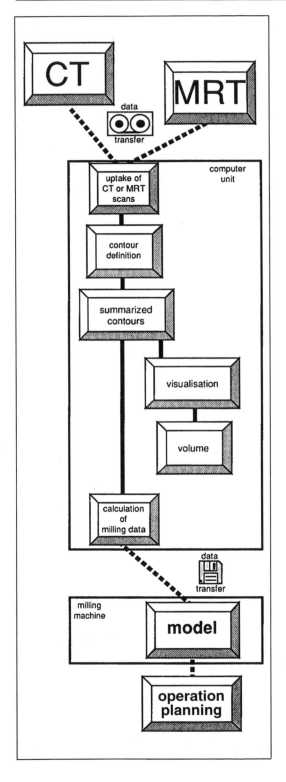

Fig. 28 Schematic view of process steps with additional integration of MRT data.

Milling Process

As specified by the computer, a block of the selected model material was cut to size manually and glued; it was then clamped to the workpiece basket of the milling machine. After transfer of the milling data to the control computer, the actual milling process was begun. The speed of the milling motor was set manually to accommodate the milling tool and model material selected. The milling process began with a coarse shaping of the raw workpiece. After a tool change, final precision milling of the model surface occurred. Upon completion of the milling process, the nonmilled sections of the workpiece, on which the model had been supported, were severed.

A custom-fitted base was furnished for each mandibular model. With the help of a special contour-finding feature of the software, a partial negative mold of the mandible could be produced. The computer-generated model base ensured a stable position of the mandibular model and the mandibular condyles, even when the "bone" was severed in one or more places.

Magnetic Resonance Tomography

Although computerized tomography is able to furnish precise images of bone structures of the skull and the mandible, the process involves the risk of radiation exposure, especially when applied repeatedly. Ultrasound echograms, at the current state of technology, still have certain shortcomings when used as basic information for three-dimensional imaging applications. When it comes to the processing of two-dimensional structures, magnetic resonance tomography avoids these disadvantages and is superior to other processes for the analysis of soft tissue structures. It does not expose the patient to ionizing radiation and can, therefore, be used (according to current research) repeatedly without risk for monitoring the success of therapy.

MRT Images

The MRT system Gyroscan S 15 made by Philips has a magnet with an operating field strength of 1.5 Tesla. The images were processed by a VAX II/750 computer using a 456-MB hard disk for data storage. Several types of coils were available for data pickup. Compared with CT, positioning of the patient is easier: without exception, patients are able to lie relaxed on their backs. The selection of the coil position was dictated by the specific objective of the examination and the location of the target slice.

Transfer of MRT Images

Since the software described in the section on Transfer of CT images had been designed specifically for the transfer and processing of CT images, a new program (MRT acquisition) had to be developed for managing the MRT images (Fig. 28). This program made it possible to feed MRT images into the main computer system and to save the MRT image data on the hard disk. By employing the same patient record format for processing the MRT images as for the ENDOPLAN program,

the latter could also be used to manage the MRT images. The patient record format included the following parameters:

a. Patient name
b. Sex
c. Date of birth
d. Internal patient ID number
e. Date of admission
f. Description of images (organ examined and type of image)

Here, some steps of the general procedure for data acquisition, contour determination, contour summation, and for visualization differ from the procedures discussed in the section on CT image handling.

There was a linear relation between the grayscales of the MRT and the grayscales of the monitor. For reasons of compatibility, the 4096 grayscale resolution of the MRT image had to be reduced to 1500 grayscales, i.e., the resolution was reduced by a factor of 2.73. This was necessary because the contour-finding section of the program did not accept values over 1500, even though the patient record format allowed a resolution from 0 to 4096.

For displaying the images on the monitor, only 250 grayscales were made available by the computer system. With the linear grayscale display, a linear relation existed between the 1500 grayscales of the original image and the 250 grayscales of the system. The special window made it possible to assign a certain grayscale range to a larger range. For example, the grayscales from 0 to 1000 were assigned to the 0 to 50 range, the grayscales from 1001 to 1400 were assigned to the 51 to 230 range, and the grayscales from 1401 to 1500 were assigned to the 231 to 250 range. That means that while resolution in the special windows was reduced by a factor of only 2.23, it dropped by a factor of 20 in the range below, and by a factor of 5.21 in the range above the special window.

The computer aided special window generation was made by calculating the grayscales that would result from a linear grayscale display. The lower value could not be too far below the value of the linear grayscale display or else the background noise would have had an excessive influence on the contours. Usually, a value between 180 and 230 could be selected as the upper limit of the special window. The colors of 251 to 256 were reserved for graphic information of ENDOPLAN (3-D program Medizin Elektronik Kiel). The initial reduction of the resolution had no influence on accuracy because the computer calculated the grayscale of the MRT image from the grayscales of the monitor display and the assignments of the special window. The range in which the special window was to be located could be selected either directly from special points of the MRT image or independently. In addition, there was the option of inverting the MRT image. The success of the special window could be monitored directly on the screen; if the results were not satisfactory, the special window could be changed as often as necessary. Following the selection of a suitable grayscale display, the transfer of the remaining image data to the system

and their storage on the hard disk were automatic.

The organizational register followed at the end of the images. The following data were extracted:

a. Type of image
b. Slice thickness
c. Distance between slices
d. Resolution of the MRT images
e. Image diameter of the MRT images

The type of image was entered in the correct location in the data register of the 3-D program. The data on slice thickness and the distance between slices were needed to establish the table position in the organizational register. The resolution and the image diameter of the MRT images were needed for determining the scale.

The following relation was then found:

$$\text{Scale} = \frac{\text{Image diameter}}{\text{Resolution}}$$

The 3-D program uses the scale as conversion factor between the contour units and the actual size of the object. The organizational registers of the individual image sequences were generated and saved on the hard disk. Then, just as with the CT data, the MRT data were processed by the 3-D program.

Utilities

The models can be used in various ways for surgical planning, as will be seen in Part II. They offer precise information on the skeletal structures of the patient. The visual rendering of the surface conditions and the opportunity to actually "manipulate" the individual three-dimensional models represents a great improvement over the previously required mental conversion of two-dimensional information to a three-dimensional image generated solely by the imagination of the experienced surgeon. The models can also be precisely measured, and their surface contours, curves, and angles can be determined and expressed numerically.

The models themselves furnish basic information on bone thickness and volumetric conditions, as needed for surgical planning. In addition, the planned surgical procedures on skeletal skull structures can be simulated on the models and, should there be unsatisfactory results, can then be repeated as often as necessary. Especially in cases with asymmetric conditions, the use of the three-dimensional models introduces new and progressive aspects to the planning of surgical procedures. If a tumor necessitates the resection of the mandible, the bone section to be removed during the operation can be located on the model surface and excised from the model. At the same time, the optimal cutting and sawing techniques for the planned procedure can be determined and practiced on the model. After studying and measuring the model surface, it is then possible to design rehabilitation plates that will be suitable for the loads and stresses exerted on a particular area. Following the contours of the model, the osteosynthesis plate, usually a prefabricated flat plate, is adapted and shaped for a perfect fit.

The firm attachment of the plates is ensured by bicortical socket head screws and special osteosynthesis screws. Again, the spatial conditions clearly reflected in the model permit ready determination of the necessary number of the screws, the position of the screw holes, and the length of the screws, all of which are dependent on the bone thickness in these areas. The precise cross-section of the mandible is manifest on the model. The correct fit of the shaped plate can be verified by trial-fitting it firmly to the milled model.

To determine shape and size of grafts for filling defects, models of the resected segment can be prepared. Beside the volume, these partial models also provided information on lost surface area in the resected area. They served as precise three-dimensional replicas of size and volume for the rehabilitation of the structural continuity.

The selected screws, the preshaped resection plate, the model of the resected segment, and all instruments were cleaned and sterilized prior to surgery. To protect the model surface against abrasion during surgery, it was necessary to seal the surface of the model of the resected segment with a heat-resistant enamel prior to sterilization.

In cases of unilateral mandibular rehabilitation, a mirror-imaging technique was used to fabricate a model with reversed sides. In combination with the true model, this mirror-image model facilitated a symmetrical rehabilitation of the mandible by providing three-dimensional information on the desired shape and size of grafts for filling in defects. The models also proved to be useful for demonstrating planned surgical procedures to patients by facilitating understanding of the various steps of the complex surgical procedure.

The average time required for the various steps in the fabrication of a model of the skull or the mandible was as follows:

a. CT scan   60 to 75 min
b. Transfer of CT data   30 min
c. Contour determination   60 min
d. Calculation of milling data   90 min
e. Transfer of the milling data
    to the milling machine and
    preparation of workpiece   10 min
f. Premilling of mandibular
    model   20 to 35 min
g. Precision-milling of
    mandibular model   3 to 4.5 h

In the time period between June 1985 and May 1991, we fabricated the following numbers of 3-D models:

Whole skull, maxilla and mandible	15
Central portion of face and maxilla	21
Mandible	40
Temporomandibular joint	11
Soft tissue structures	2

3. Case Studies

To illustrate the possibilities offered by three-dimensional model fabrication in oral and maxillofacial surgery, several cases are presented. In principle, planning based on three-dimensional technology is possible with and without the fabrication of models.

Planning without Model Fabrication

Case 1 Meningo-encephalocystocele
(Figs. 29 to 40)

The newborn child shown in Fig. 29 was born with a meningoencephalocystocele. A CT scan (Fig. 30) indicated portions of the brain at a central level of the bulbus. The visualization (Figs. 31 and 32) showed two ruptures in the area of the supraorbital bulges. The open fontanelles did not permit the fabrication of a solid three-dimensional model; thus, surgical planning was based on the information provided by visualization alone. After aspiration of the cele (Fig. 33) and transcranial approach (Fig. 34) were performed, the dural defects were dissected and closed (Fig. 35).

Step by step (Figs. 36 to 38), the medial eye angle, the glabella, and the nose were reconstructed using available soft tissue from the facial area. The subsequent development of the child, observed during a check-up 17 days after surgery (Fig. 39) and again one year after surgery (Fig. 40), was proof of the satisfactory result of the procedure.

Planning with Model Fabrication

Case 2 Synostosis of the Metopic Suture
(Figs. 41 to 54)

The boy shown in Fig. 41 showed flattening of the left cheek and temple region that could not be correlated radiographically with any pathological finding (Fig. 42). A CT scan at the upper orbital level (Fig. 43) showed a distinct asymmetry in the area of the lateral orbital wall. This could be considered a position-linked asymmetry because of the side difference in the medial fossa of the skull base.

Contour summations (Figs. 44 and 45) gave no hint of asymmetrical skeletal features in the clinically relevant region. Visualization was performed. Neither frontal (Fig. 46) nor dorsal (Fig. 47) views gave additional information. Comparison, how-

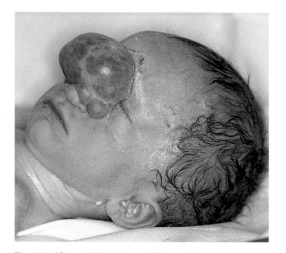

Fig. 29 (Case 1) Newborn child with frontal meningo-encephalocystocele.

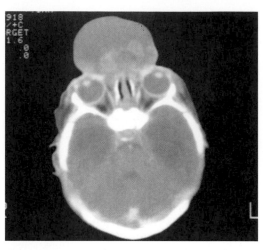

Fig. 30 (Case 1) CT scan at a central level of the bulbus.

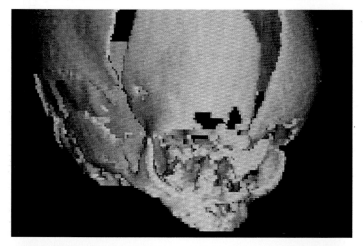

Fig. 31 (Case 1) Visualization displays two supraorbital ruptures.

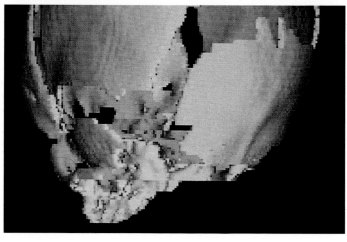

Fig. 32 (Case 1) Visualization displays one supraorbital rupture (temporo-dorsal view).

ever, of the right lateral visualization (45 degrees) to the left lateral visualization (Figs. 48 and 49) revealed a shallow metopic suture on the left lateral side. At first glance, even a frontal view of the 3-D model (Fig. 50) and the exarticulated mandible (Fig. 51) did not permit a clear diagnosis.

Only the exarticulation of the mandible from the model and a caudal examination of the base of the skull revealed the hypoplasia of the left zygoma and the zygomatic arch (Fig. 52). Early synostosis of the left metopic suture with simultaneous underdevelopment of the zygoma and the zygomatic arch was diagnosed. Figs. 53 and 54 permit comparison of both sides of the clinical and skeletal views from a lateral perspective. It became clear that the increased distance between the base of the nose and the lateral corner of the eye had skeletal causes. To date, craniofacial surgery has not been indicated. If it were, a model would permit precise planning of the procedure.

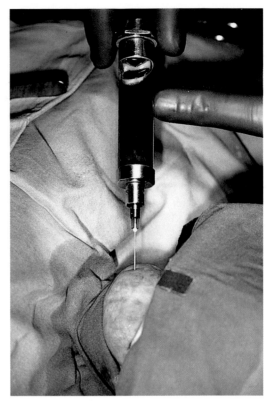

Fig. 33 (Case 1) Aspiration of liquid from meningo-encephalocystocele.

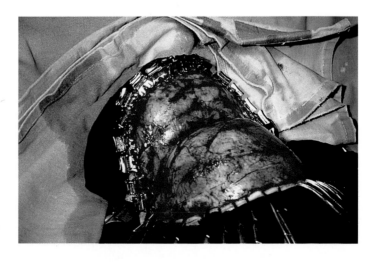

Fig. 34 (Case 1) Transcranial approach.

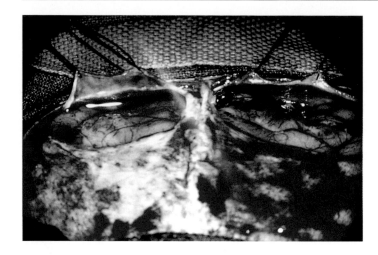

Fig. 35 (Case 1) Intraoperative display of dura perforation before duraplasty.
(Surgery performed by H. Klinge, M.D., Dept. of Neurosurgery, University Hospital, Kiel, Germany.)

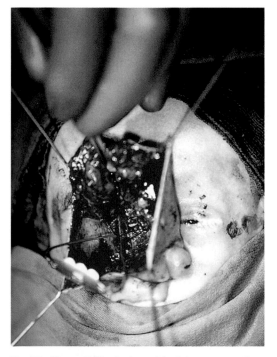

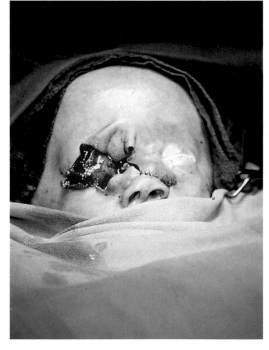

Fig. 36 (Case 1) Beginning of facial reconstruction.
(Surgery performed by Prof. F. Härle, M.D., D.M.D.)

Fig. 37 (Case 1) Adaptation of redundant material.

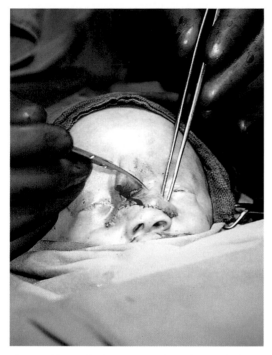

Fig. 38 (Case 1) Final phase of midface soft tissue reconstruction.

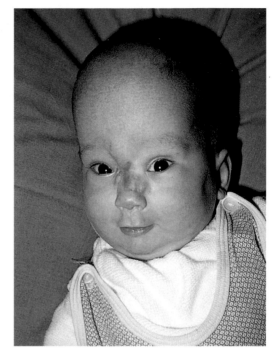

Fig. 39 (Case 1) Appearance 17 days after surgery.

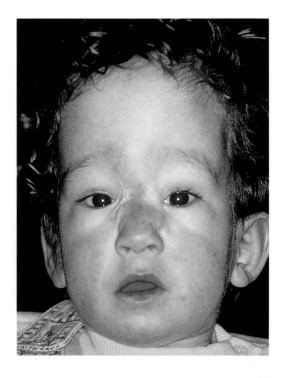

Fig. 40 (Case 1) Appearance one year after surgery.

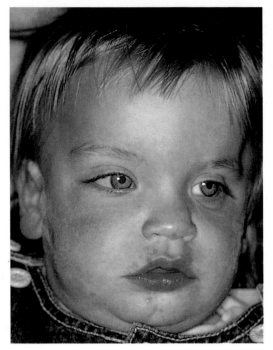

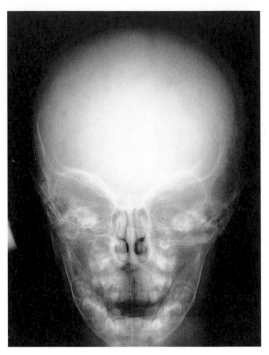

Fig. 41 (Case 2) A two-year-old boy shows synostosis of the left metopic suture.

Fig. 42 (Case 2) Radiograph shows no pathologic findings.

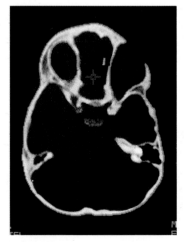

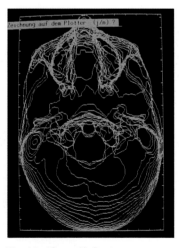

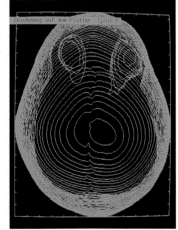

Fig. 43 (Case 2) Contoured CT scan at the upper orbital level shows distinct asymmetry of the lateral orbital wall.

Fig. 44 (Case 2) Contour summation of the skull base shows no asymmetry.

Fig. 45 (Case 2) Contour summation of the calotte shows mild asymmetry.

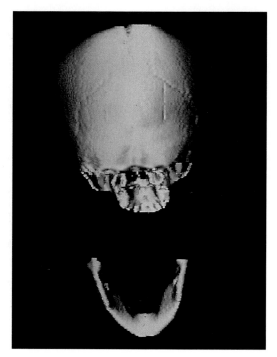

Fig. 46 (Case 2) Visualization (frontal view) with mathematically exarticulated mandible.

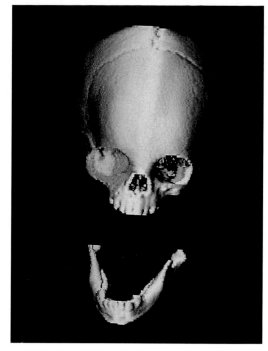

Fig. 47 (Case 2) Visualization (dorsal view) with mathematically exarticulated mandible.

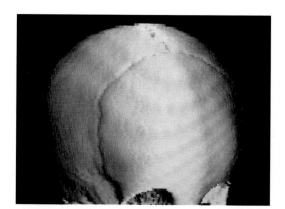

Fig. 48 (Case 2) Right lateral visualization (45 degrees) shows visible sutures.

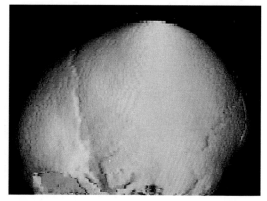

Fig. 49 (Case 2) Left lateral visualization shows sutures that seem diffuse and shallow.

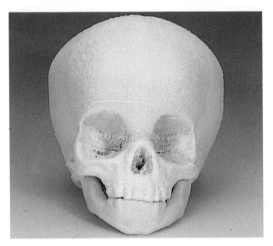

Fig. 50 (Case 2) 3-D Styrodur model of skull on a frontal view shows no pathologic findings.

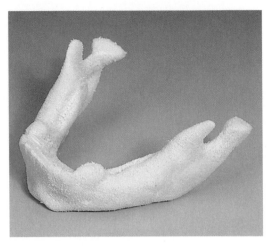

Fig. 51 (Case 2) 3-D Styrodur model of mandible shows no pathologic findings.

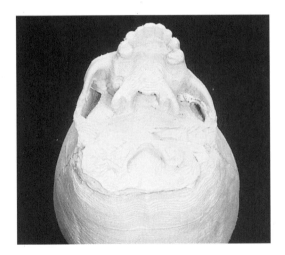

Fig. 52 (Case 2) 3-D Styrodur model of skull (mandible removed) on a caudal view shows distinct hypoplasia of left zygoma and zygomatic arch.

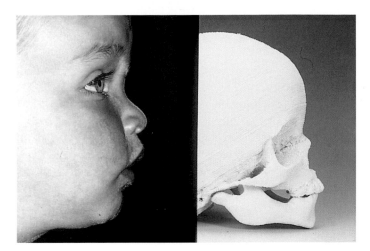

Fig. 53 (Case 2) Comparison of right lateral views: clinical vs model.

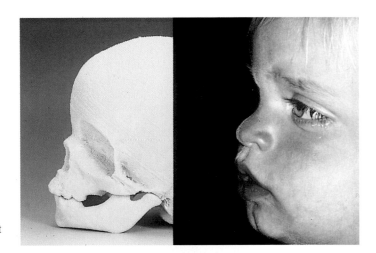

Fig. 54 (Case 2) Comparison of left lateral views: clinical vs model.

Case 3 Crouzon's Disease
(Figs. 55 to 64)

A two-year-old girl with typical Crouzon disease symptoms is shown in a clinical profile in Fig. 55 and in a right lateral radiograph in Fig. 56. Visualization (Fig. 57) permitted views from several sides (Fig. 58), and mathematical subtractions of the right temporal calotte produced a view inside the cranium (Fig. 59). After rough and smooth grinding (Fig. 60) the completed model was studied (Figs. 61 and 62).

A 3-D surgical simulation using Marchac's method (1978) was performed. Osteotomy lines were drawn (Fig. 63) and, after exchange of calottal parts, potential miniplate osteosynthesis was modeled (Fig. 64).

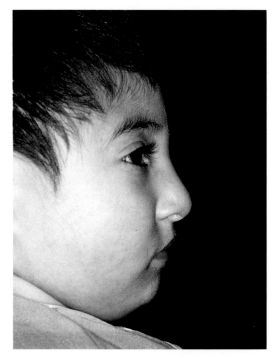

Fig. 55 (Case 3) Two-year-old patient with Crouzon's disease (right lateral view).

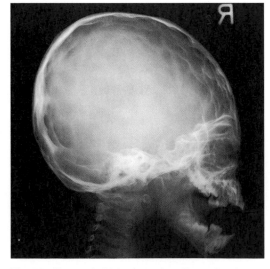

Fig. 56 (Case 3) Right lateral radiograph of skull shows lateral "impressiones digitorum" all over the calotte.

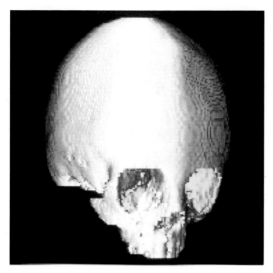

Fig. 57 (Case 3) Half-profile visualization.

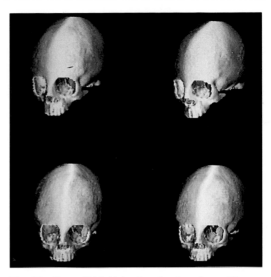

Fig. 58 (Case 3) Multiple visualizations from different perspectives.

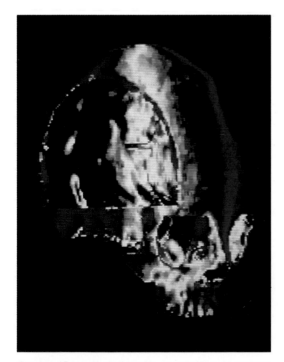

Fig. 59 (Case 3) Half-profile visualization in multiple colors, with mathematical subtraction of the right part of the calotte.

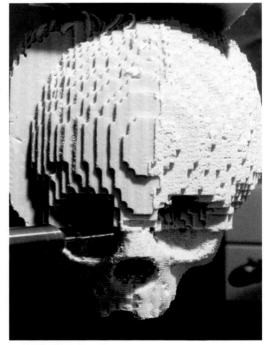

Fig. 60 (Case 3) Rough and smooth grinding during model fabrication.

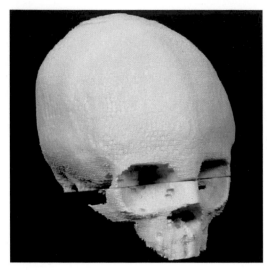

Fig. 61 (Case 3) 3-D right lateral model (45 degrees).

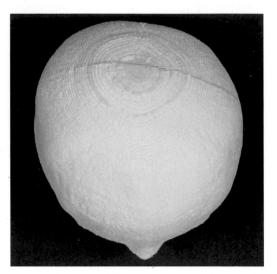

Fig. 62 (Case 3) 3-D cranial model shows mild dorsoparietal asymmetry at left.

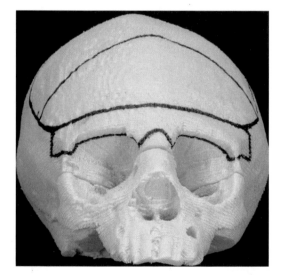

Fig. 63 (Case 3) 3-D model with osteotomy lines drawn in.

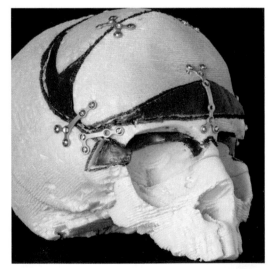

Fig. 64 (Case 3) 3-D model shows surgical simulation (Marchac's method) and osteosynthesis material in place.

Case 4. Hemifacial Dysplasia
(Figs. 65 to 75)

Correction of facial asymmetries caused by both skeletal and soft tissue deficiencies can be planned and realized using 3-D technologies. The patient shown in Figs. 65 to 75 had undergone skeletal surgery prior to requesting additional soft tissue surgery. The desired result was visualized in a standard patient information 2-D program (Figs. 65 and 66), and in a 3-D program (Fig. 67).

The 3-D model (Fig. 68) was symmetrically enhanced using a model of missing soft tissue structures (Fig. 69). This enabled a volumetric 3-D assessment of the placement and inflation of the tissue expander (Fig. 70) and of the size of the microvascular pedicellate omentum majus transplant (Fig. 71).

The preoperative (Fig. 72) and postoperative (Fig. 73) CT scans allow comparison of the desired result with the actual situation achieved by transplantation. Figs. 74 and 75 show clinical appearances of the patient before and after surgery.

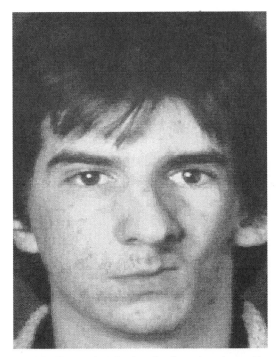

Fig. 65 (Case 4) 2-D visualization of patient with hemifacial dysplasia.

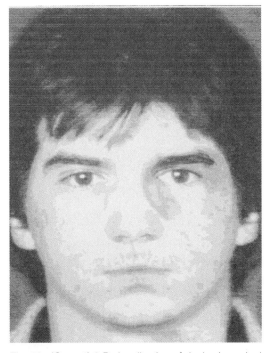

Fig. 66 (Case 4) 2-D visualization of desired surgical result.

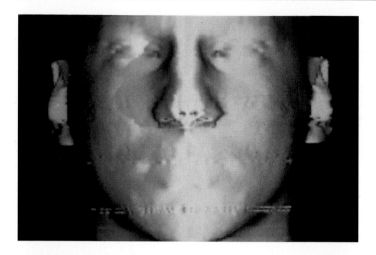

Fig. 67 (Case 4) 3-D visualization of desired surgical result.

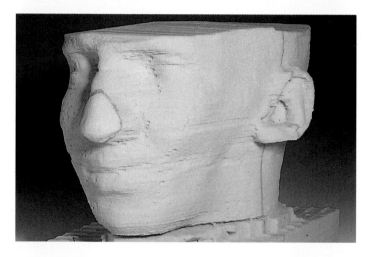

Fig. 68 (Case 4) 3-D model of preoperative soft tissue situation.

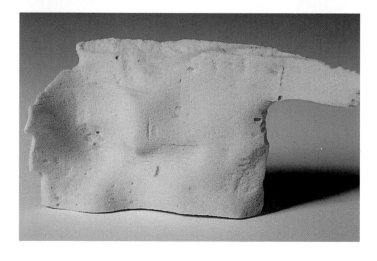

Fig. 69 (Case 4) 3-D model revealing absent soft tissue structures.

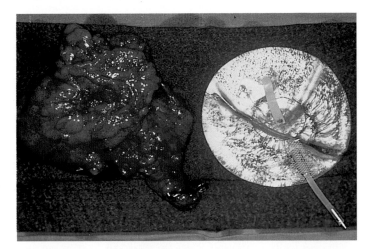

Fig. 70 (Case 4) Intraoperative situation:
(left) removed tissue expander,
(right) microvascular pedicellate
omentum majus transplant.

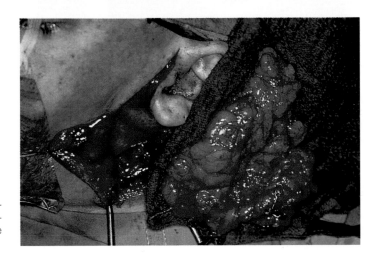

Fig. 71 (Case 4) Intraoperative situation: pre-auricular cut for placement of microvascular pedicellate omentum majus transplant.

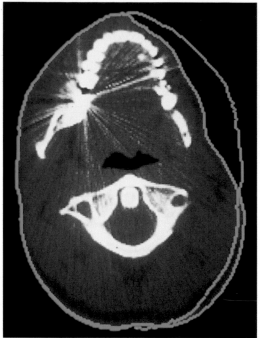

Fig. 72 (Case 4) Preoperative CT scan shows desired soft tissue contour (mirror technique placement).

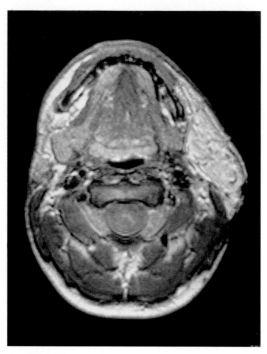

Fig. 73 (Case 4) Postoperative MRT scan shows result of surgical soft tissue contouring.

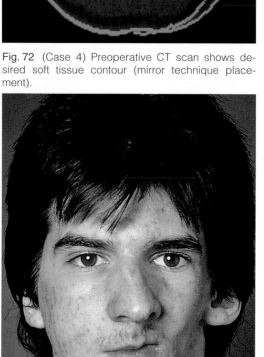

Fig. 74 (Case 4) Appearance before surgery.

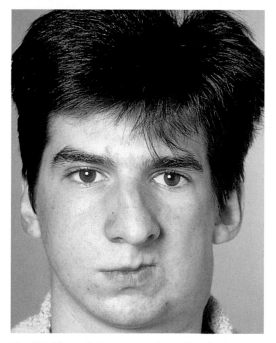

Fig. 75 (Case 4) Appearance 6 months after surgery. Patient planned to undergo further surgeries.

Case 5 Bimaxillary Surgical Procedure

(Figs. 76 to 83)

Using an articulator, the skull model and the maxilla were precisely positioned with the help of the face-bow (Figs. 76 to 78). The plaster models were used in the styrodur models in order to obtain precise occlusal information.

After the mandible was adjusted and the centric splint inserted, right and left positioning plates were installed and attached with two screws each to the zygoma and laterally to the mandible in the area of its angle (Fig. 79). Photographs taken during surgery were only partially successful in showing the position of the plates (Fig. 80).

Therefore, the 3-D model was ideally suited to explain and demonstrate the steps of the surgical procedure. The lateral view (Fig. 81) shows that the maxilla is already osteotomized in the Le Fort I plane and has been moved up. The considerably more-voluminous splint indicates the new maxillomandibular relation. The mandible remained in the original position since the position of the positioning plates was not changed; the relations in the TMJ area also remained unchanged.

Following the fixation of the maxilla with miniplate osteosyntheses, the mandible was split sagittally on both sides, and the central section of the mandible was fixed in the desired occlusal position by means of the third, definitive splint, which was fabricated prior to surgery. The lateral segments of the mandible carrying the TMJ remained, again, in their original positions (Fig. 82).

The positioning plates were not removed until the segments on the mandible had been fixed in place by three adjusting screws on both sides. The surgical procedure ended with the bimaxillary 3-D block in the desired position, while the position of the TMJs remained unchanged (Fig. 83).

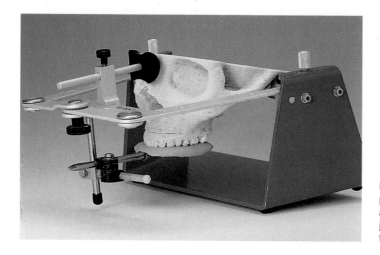

Fig. 76 (Case 5) Model of skull and plaster model of teeth and maxillary alveolar process, individually adjusted in the SAM apparatus with the face-bow.

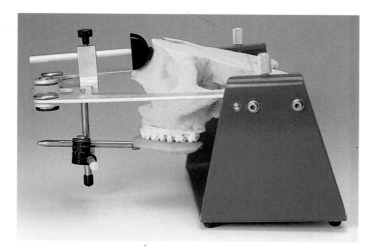

Fig. 77 (Case 5) Left lateral view of model in SAM apparatus.

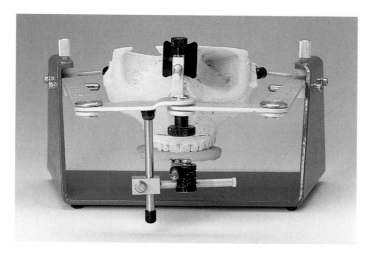

Fig. 78 (Case 5) Frontal view of model in SAM apparatus.

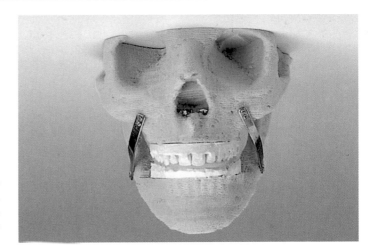

Fig. 79 (Case 5) Demonstration of bimaxillary surgery using a 3-D model that reflects Class II malocclusion and shows splint and positioning plates in place.

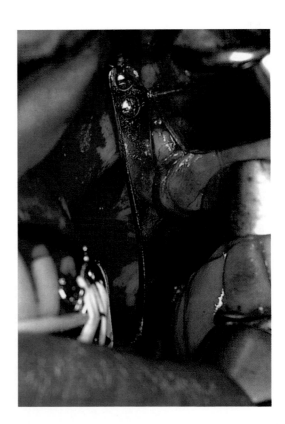

Fig. 80 (Case 5) Upper end of the positioning plate on the zygoma is visible; lower end at the mandibular angle is out of camera view.

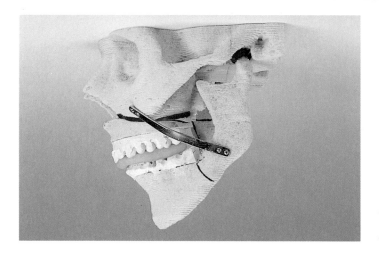

Fig. 81 (Case 5) Model shows maxilla osteotomized and cranialized, splint and positioning plates in place, and mandible remaining in original position.

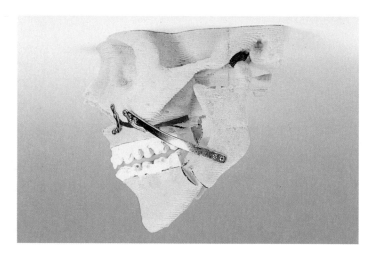

Fig. 82 (Case 5) Model shows maxilla osteotomized and, with positioning plates in place, set in the correct occlusal position in the splint.

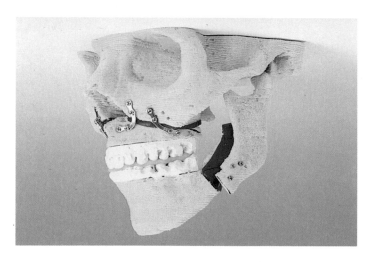

Fig. 83 (Case 5) Model indicates that after surgery, the position of the TMJ would remain unchanged.

Case 6 Computerized Tomography and Magnetic Resonance Tomography of the TMJ (Figs. 84 to 90)

Fig. 84 shows differently scaled polyurethane models of the right TMJ region. Depending on the contour limits, individual portions could be enlarged.

Fig. 85 shows the MRT scan of a left TMJ with prolapsed articular disk. After contouring of the disk (Fig. 86), even this cartilaginous structure and its relation to the condyle could be recreated in the 3-D model (Figs. 87 to 90).

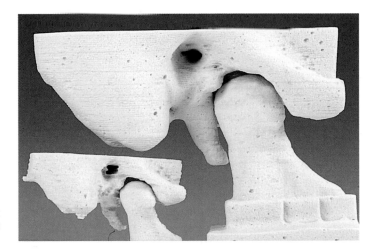

Fig. 84 (Case 6) Models of the right TMJ: 1:1 scale (left) and 1:2 scale (right).

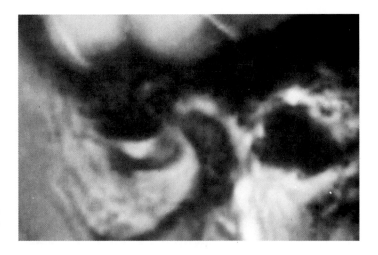

Fig. 85 (Case 6) MRT scan of the left TMJ shows prolapse of articular disk (closed-mouth position).

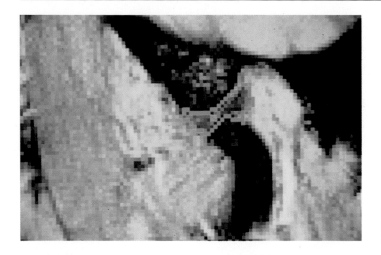

Fig. 86 (Case 6) Contouring of the articular disk (green line) (open-mouth position).

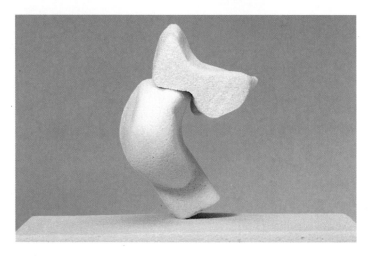

Fig. 87 (Case 6) 3-D model of condyle and disk (1:3 scale) (closed-mouth position).

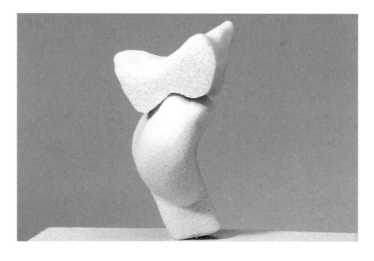

Fig. 88 (Case 6) 3-D model of condyle and disk (1:3 scale) (open-mouth position).

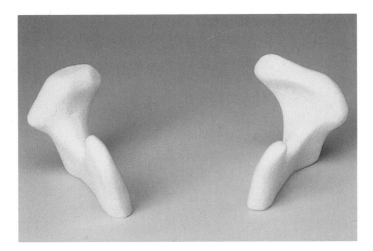

Fig. 89 (Case 6) Flattening of the lateral part of the right temporo-mandibular joint is evident.

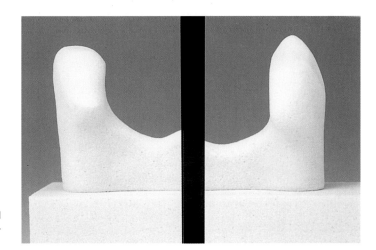

Fig. 90 (Case 6) 3-D model lateral view comparison: notice the irregular shape of the right condyle.

Demonstration of Surgical Technique

Case 7 Traumatology
(Figs. 91 to 100)

So far, primary traumatologic aspects have been evaluated only via visualization. Fig. 91 shows a fracture of the right zygoma with a multiple fracture of the orbital floor and a fracture of the facial sinus wall. Fig. 92 shows a multiple fracture of the frontal sinus. The visualization was used for the demonstration, since the need for immediate primary traumatologic care left insufficient time for fabricating a model prior to surgery.

3-D technology is particularly suitable for surgical planning and simulation in secondary traumatologic cases. Fig. 99 shows a patient who suffered severe comminuted lower- and mid-face fractures as a result of a car accident. The drawings (Figs. 93 and 94) represent traditional 2-D surgical planning. 3-D simulation of surgery and intra-operative position as seen from the same perspective in Figs. 95 and 96 show the millimeter-precise planning and execution (Fig. 97 and 98) of the procedure.

Photographs of the patient (Figs. 99 and 100) taken both before and after a late secondary traumatologic surgical treatment convey some impression of the value of this technology.

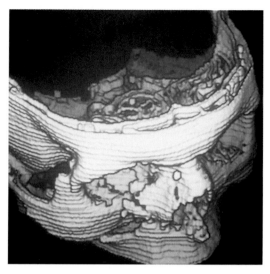

Fig. 91 (Case 7) Visualization of a fracture of the right zygoma.

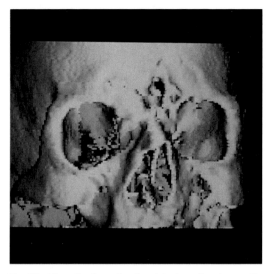

Fig. 92 Visualization of a frontal sinus fracture with defect.

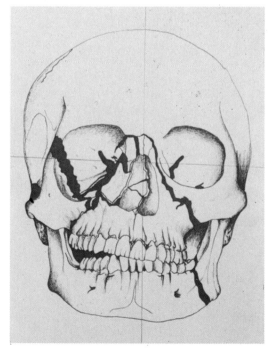

Fig. 93 (Case 7) Conventional 2-D drawing of a centrolateral comminuted midfacial trauma and fracture of the lower jaw. (Dr. B. Hammer)

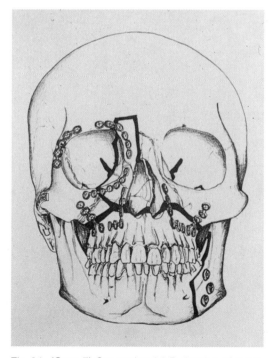

Fig. 94 (Case 7) Conventional 2-D drawing of surgical plan. (Dr. B. Hammer)

69

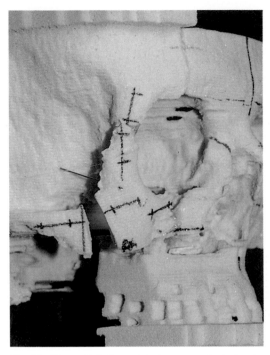

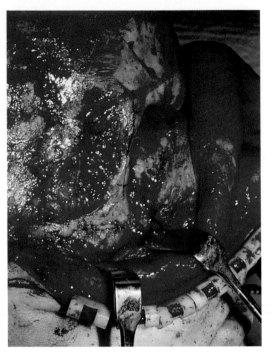

Fig. 95 (Case 7) 3-D model shows surgical simulation.

Fig. 96 (Case 7) Intraoperative situation (from a similar perspective as that seen in Fig. 95): notice the transfer of screw points (landmarks).

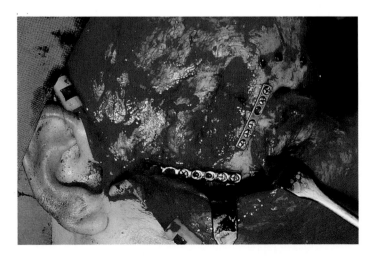

Fig. 97 (Case 7) Intraoperative situation after osteosynthesis.
(Surgery performed by B. Hammer, M.D., D.M.D., Dept. of Reconstructive Surgery, University Hospital, Basel, Switzerland.)

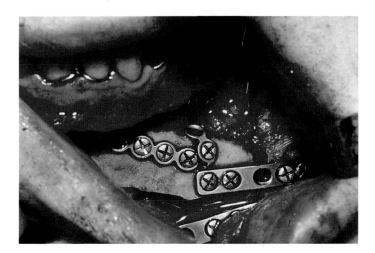

Fig. 98 (Case 7) Intraoral approach.

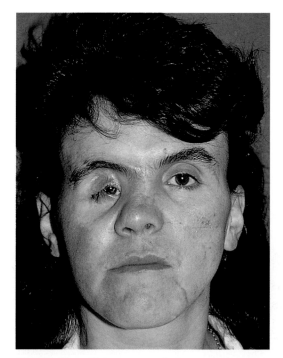

Fig. 99 (Case 7) Appearance before surgery.

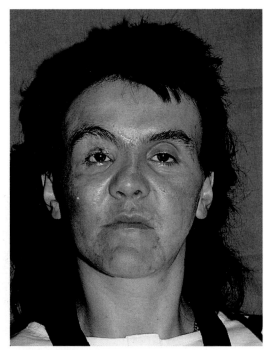

Fig. 100 (Case 7) Appearance after surgery.

Case 8 Preprosthetic Surgery (Figs. 101 to 109)

Following 3-D planning, asymmetrical conditions in the area of the edentulous mandible can be corrected through preprosthetic measures. Fig. 101 shows the 3-D model of an asymmetrically atrophied mandible (greater deficit on left) and the compensation achieved with an appropriately shaped vicryl mesh tube filled with hydroxylapatite. The findings during surgery (Fig. 102) confirmed the flattening in the area of the left vestibule.

Immediately after the end of the operation, the same level was reached on both sides (Fig. 103). Preoperative and postoperative radiographs (Figs. 104 and 105) showed the result achieved after 3-D planning.

According to our expectations, the results of the axial CT scans compared those of the coronal slices (Fig. 106). Here, it was important that the edentulous patients kept the mandible absolutely motionless. An intraoral splint was helpful.

In some cases, it is difficult to use implants for preprosthetic surgery in an edentulous mandible since an incorrectly seated implant will perforate the basal cortical bone (Fig. 107). Here, the 3-D model allowed a determination of the exact size of the implant and precise drilling and insertion directions, so that the implant could be firmly placed and surrounded by cortical bone on all sides (Fig. 108). This, however, may not always be the ideal position for the suprastructure (Fig. 109).

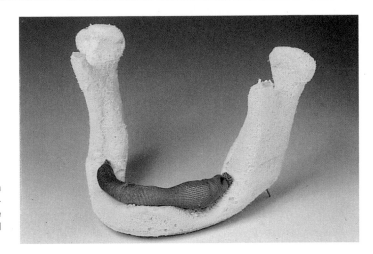

Fig. 101 (Case 8) 3-D model of an asymmetrically atrophied edentulous mandible shows build-up of the ridge with a vicryl mesh tube filled with hydroxylapatite.

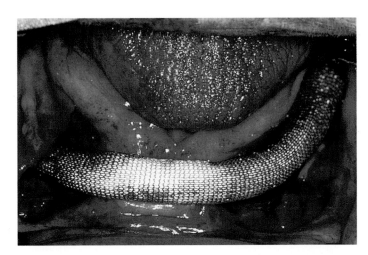

Fig. 102 (Case 8) Intraoperative situation of symmetrically filled vicryl mesh tube shows the low level at left lateral surface of mandible.

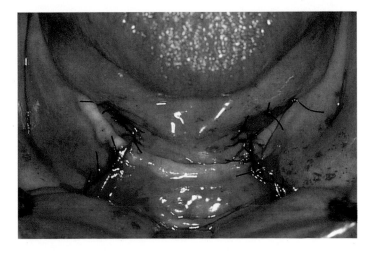

Fig. 103 (Case 8) Postoperative situation shows an even level on left and right lateral surfaces.

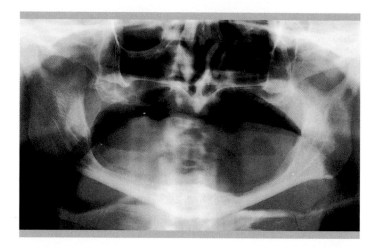

Fig. 104 (Case 8) Preoperative radiograph shows asymmetrical atrophy of mandible.

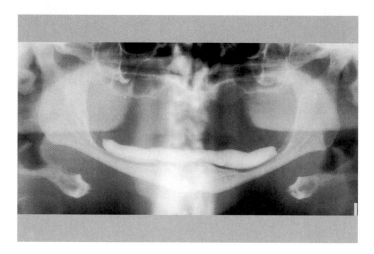

Fig. 105 (Case 8) Postoperative radiograph shows vicryl mesh tube in place.

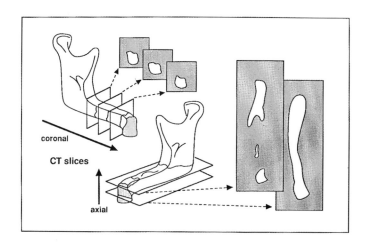

Fig. 106 Information from CT scans taken in different scanning axes on edentulous mandibles in the course of preprosthetic planning.

Fig. 107 Incorrectly seated implant in model of an edentulous mandible.

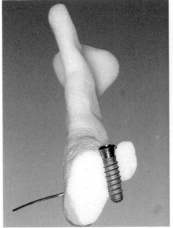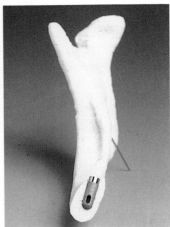

Fig. 108 Correctly seated implant in model of an edentulous mandible.

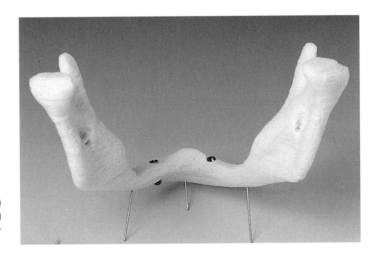

Fig. 109 3-D model (dorsal view) shows left implant to be perforating the bone and right implant to be surrounded by cortical bone.

Case 9 Angle Class II Malocclusion

(Figs. 110 to 121;
see also Figs. 76 to 83)

Clinical pictures and radiographs show a patient with Class II malocclusion, whose models were presented in Case 5 (Figs. 76 to 83).

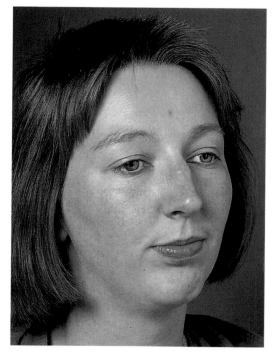

Fig. 110 (Cases 5 and 9) Appearance before surgery (right lateral view, 45 degrees).

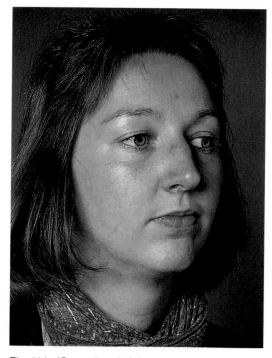

Fig. 111 (Cases 5 and 9) Appearance one year after bimaxillary osteotomy (right lateral view, 45 degrees).

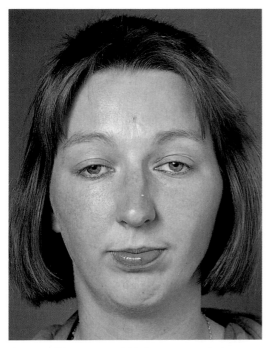

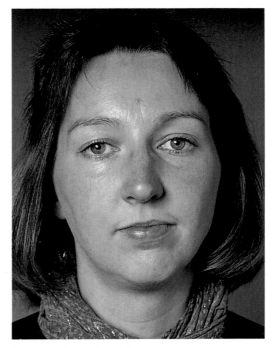

Fig. 112 (Cases 5 and 9) Appearance before surgery.

Fig. 113 (Cases 5 and 9) Appearance one year after bimaxillary osteotomy.

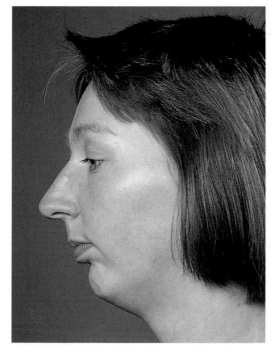

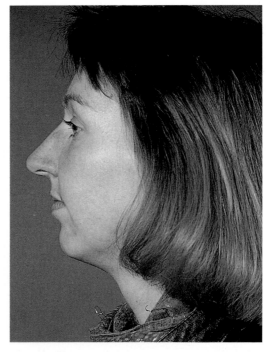

Fig. 114 (Cases 5 and 9) Appearance before surgery (left lateral view).

Fig. 115 (Cases 5 and 9) Appearance one year after bimaxillary osteotomy (left lateral view).

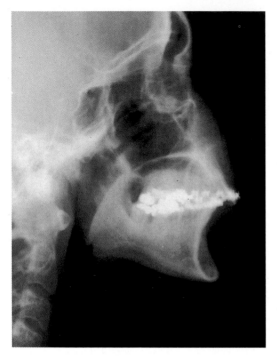

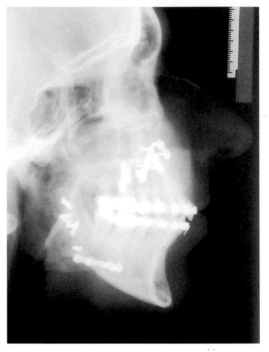

Fig. 116 (Cases 5 and 9) Preoperative right lateral skull radiograph.

Fig. 117 (Cases 5 and 9) Postoperative right lateral skull radiograph.

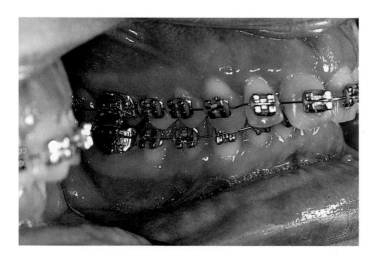

Fig. 118 (Cases 5 and 9) Preoperative occlusion (right lateral view).

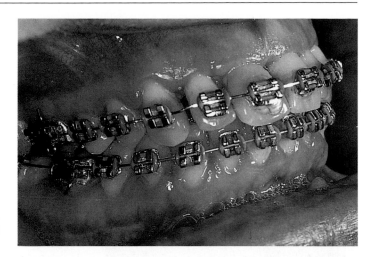

Fig. 119 (Cases 5 and 9) Post-operative occlusion (right lateral view).

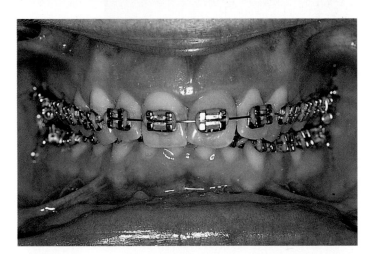

Fig. 120 (Cases 5 and 9) Pre-operative occlusion (frontal view).

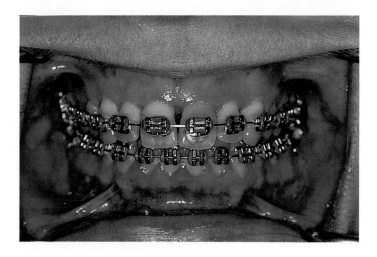

Fig. 121 (Cases 5 and 9) Post-operative occlusion (frontal view).

Case 10 Angle Class III Malocclusion
(Figs. 122 to 170)

This case concerned a patient with a Class III malocclusion. The therapy involved a bimaxillary surgical procedure that established the correct occlusion by moving the maxilla forward and the mandible back. There were no lateral asymmetries.

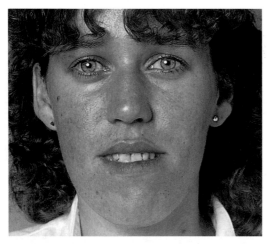

Fig. 122 (Case 10) Patient with Class III malocclusion before surgery.

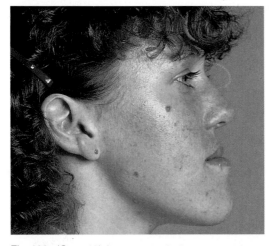

Fig. 123 (Case 10) Appearance before surgery (right lateral view).

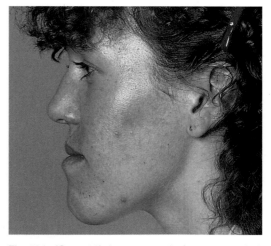

Fig. 124 (Case 10) Appearance before surgery (left lateral view).

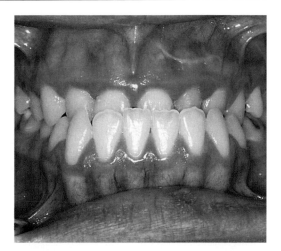

Fig. 125 (Case 10) Preoperative occlusion (frontal view).

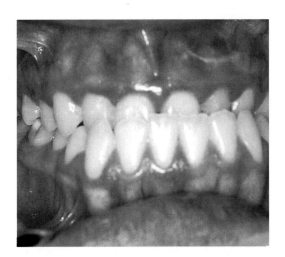

Fig. 126 (Case 10) Preoperative occlusion (right frontal view).

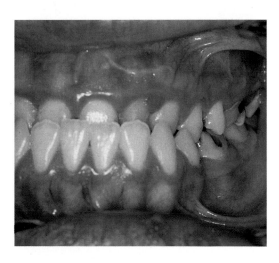

Fig. 127 (Case 10) Preoperative occlusion (left frontal view).

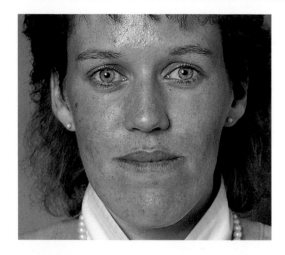

Fig. 128 (Case 10) Appearance before surgery but after orthodontic treatment (shaping of the arches of upper and lower jaw, independent of present occlusion).

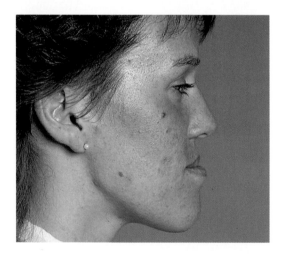

Fig. 129 (Case 10) Appearance before surgery (right lateral view).

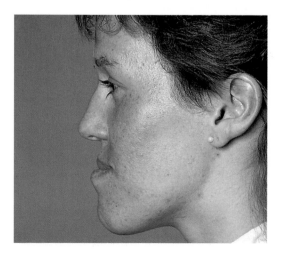

Fig. 130 (Case 10) Appearance before surgery (after orthodontic treatment) (left lateral view). Notice distinct pouting of the lower lip due to protrusion of the lower front teeth.

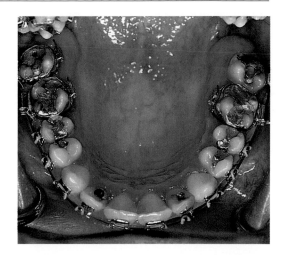

Fig. 131 (Case 10) Preoperative situation of ortho-dontically shaped upper jaw.

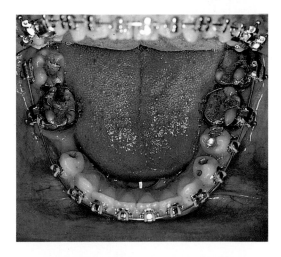

Fig. 132 (Case 10) Preoperative situation of ortho-dontically shaped lower jaw.

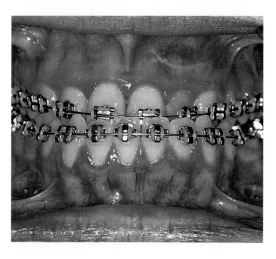

Fig. 133 (Case 10) Preoperative occlusion (frontal view) after orthodontic treatment.

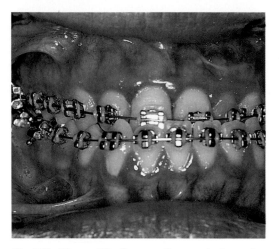

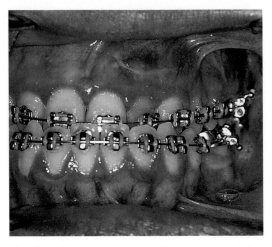

Fig. 134 (Case 10) Preoperative occlusion after orthodontic treatment (right frontal view).

Fig. 135 (Case 10) Preoperative occlusion after orthodontic treatment (left frontal view).

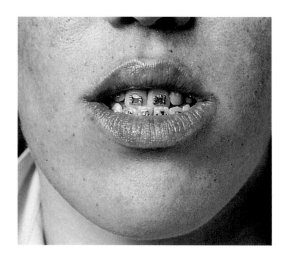

Fig. 136 (Case 10) Appearance before surgery but after orthodontic treatment. Lip closure is incomplete when facial mimic muscles are relaxed.

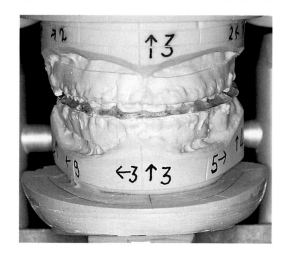

Fig. 137 (Case 10) Conventional planning of surgical intervention with SAM articulator (frontal view).

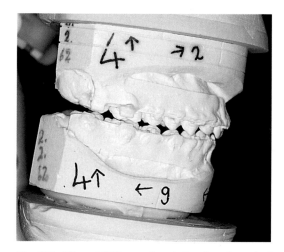

Fig. 138 (Case 10) Conventional planning of surgical intervention with SAM articulator (right lateral view).

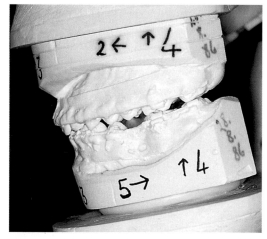

Fig. 139 (Case 10) Conventional planning of surgical intervention with SAM articulator (left lateral view).

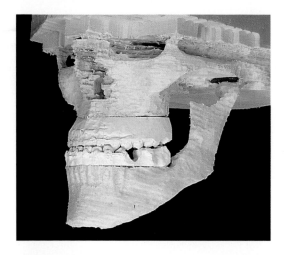

Fig. 140 (Case 10) 3-D model before surgical simulation.

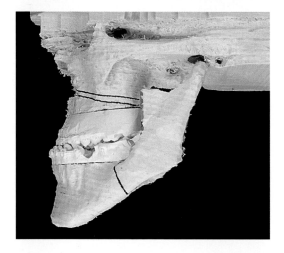

Fig. 141 (Case 10) 3-D model with osteotomy lines drawn in (left lateral view).

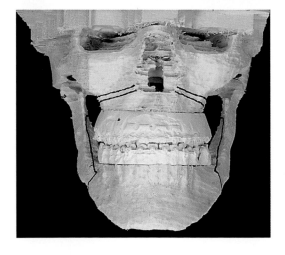

Fig. 142 (Case 10) 3-D model with osteotomy lines drawn in (frontal view).

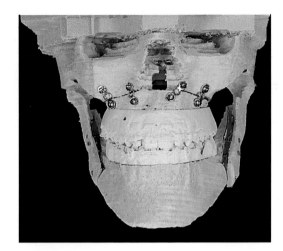

Fig. 143 (Case 10) 3-D model of surgical simulation (frontal view).

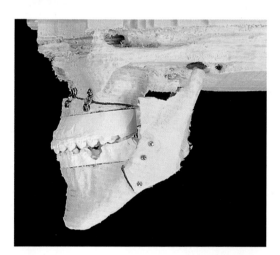

Fig. 144 (Case 10) 3-D model of surgical simulation (left lateral view).

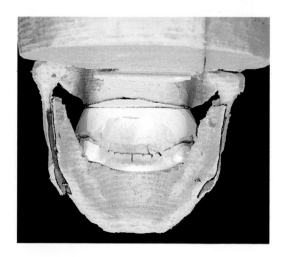

Fig. 145 (Case 10) 3-D model of surgical simulation (dorsal view). Repositioned distal portions of the interior lower jaw fragments required resection.

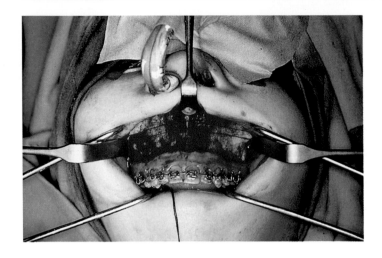

Fig. 146 (Case 10) Intraoperative situation: maxillary osteotomy, Le Fort I.

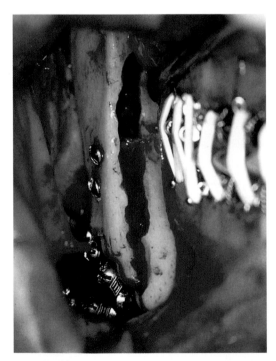

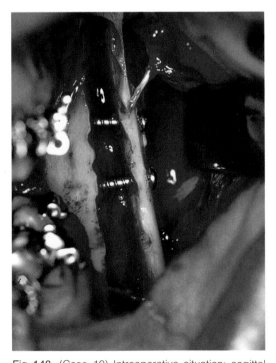

Fig. 147 (Case 10) Intraoperative situation: sagittal split procedure of right mandible, with additional implantation of an osteosynthesis miniplate to stabilize a fractured lateral segment.

Fig. 148 (Case 10) Intraoperative situation: sagittal split procedure of left mandible, with osteosynthesis screws inserted.

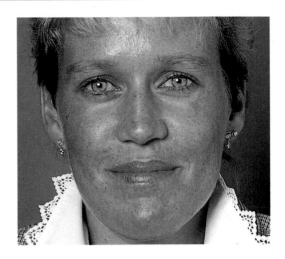

Fig. 149 (Case 10) Appearance two years after surgery.

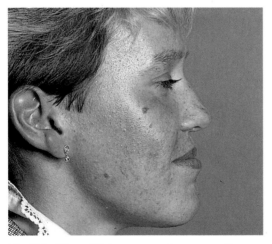

Fig. 150 (Case 10) Appearance two years after surgery (right lateral view).

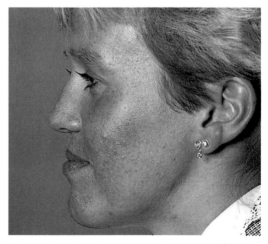

Fig. 151 (Case 10) Appearance two years after surgery (left lateral view).

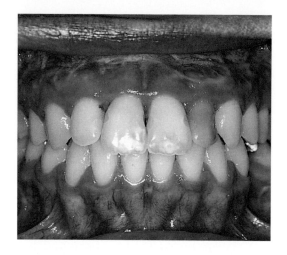

Fig. 152 (Case 10) Postoperative occlusion (frontal view).

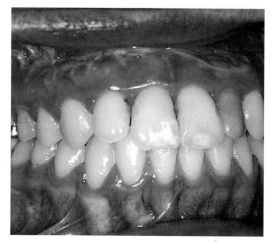

Fig. 153 (Case 10) Postoperative occlusion (right frontal view).

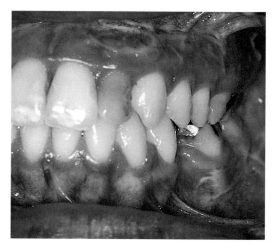

Fig. 154 (Case 10) Postoperative occlusion (left frontal view).

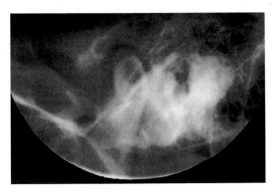

Fig. 155 (Case 10) Postoperative radiographic control of the left TMJ (closed-mouth view).

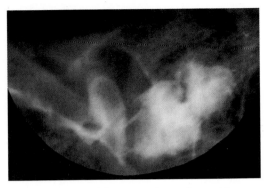

Fig. 156 (Case 10) Postoperative radiographic control of the left TMJ (open-mouth view).

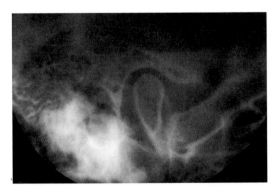

Fig. 157 (Case 10) Postoperative radiographic control of the right TMJ (closed-mouth view).

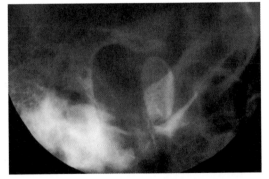

Fig. 158 (Case 10) Postoperative radiographic control of the right TMJ (open-mouth view).

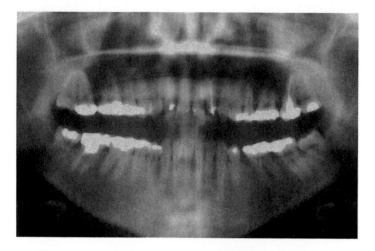

Fig. 159 (Case 10) Preoperative panoramic radiograph.

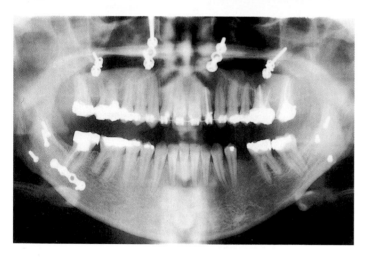

Fig. 160 (Case 10) Panoramic radiograph of situation six months after surgery, before removal of osteosynthesis material.

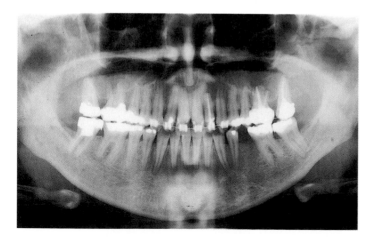

Fig. 161 (Case 10) Panoramic radiograph of situation two years after surgery.

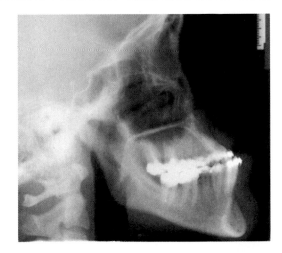

Fig. 162 (Case 10) Preoperative right lateral cephalometric radiograph.

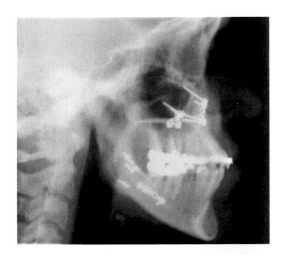

Fig. 163 (Case 10) Right lateral cephalometric radiograph of situation six months after surgery.

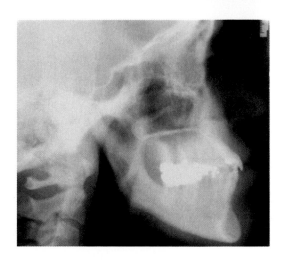

Fig. 164 (Case 10) Right lateral cephalometric radiograph of situation two years after surgery.

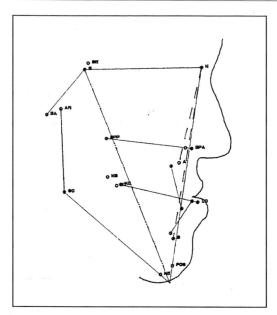

Fig. 165 (Case 10) Preoperative 2-D cephalometric analysis.

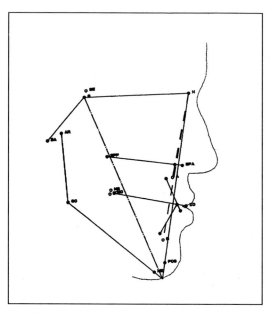

Fig. 166 (Case 10) Postoperative 2-D cephalometric analysis.

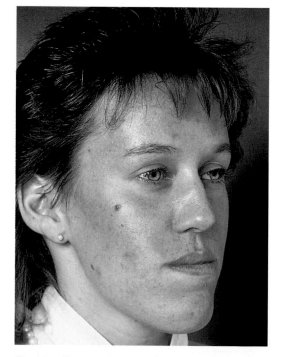

Fig. 167 (Case 10) Class III malocclusion before surgery.

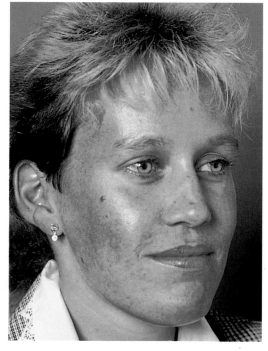

Fig. 168 (Case 10) Appearance after surgery.

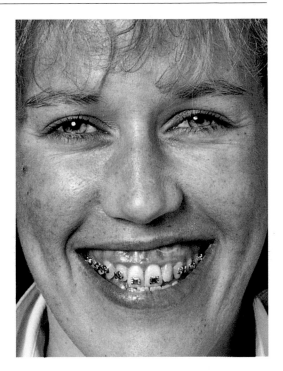

Fig. 169 (Case 10) "Gummy smile" of Class III mal-occlusion before surgery.

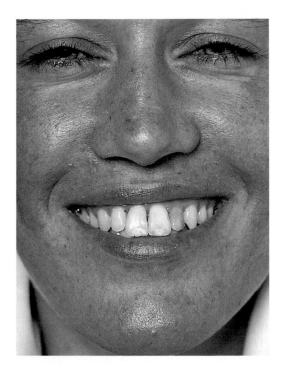

Fig. 170 (Case 10) Appearance when smiling (after surgery).

Case 11 Cleft Lip and Palate Combined with Mandibular Prognathism
(Figs. 171 to 194)

Inherited mandibular prognathism developed in an adolescent (Figs. 171 and 172) with congenital unilateral cleft lip and alveolar palate cleft (see photographs of grandfather, Fig. 173; and father, Fig. 174; progenia vera).

After visualization (Figs. 175 and 176), traditional cast model planning (Fig. 177), 3-D model planning (Figs. 178 and 179), and surgical simulation on the model (Figs. 180 and 181), the patient underwent a bimaxillary surgical intervention using a free iliac crest graft in the upper jaw (Fig. 182).

Figs. 183–194 illustrate preoperative and postoperative situations in direct comparison, using clinical photographs.

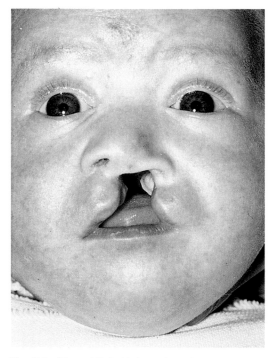

Fig. 171 (Case 11) At birth, patient shows complete unilateral cleft lip, alveolus, and palate.

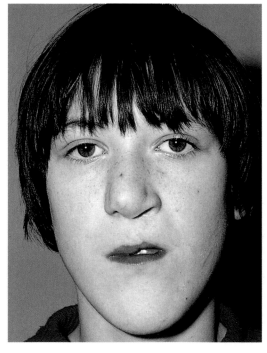

Fig. 172 (Case 11) At 10 years, patient shows result of primary closure of the cleft and exhibits beginning mandibular prognathism.

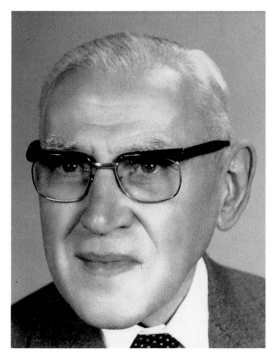

Fig. 173 (Case 11) The patient's grandfather exhibited marked prognathism.

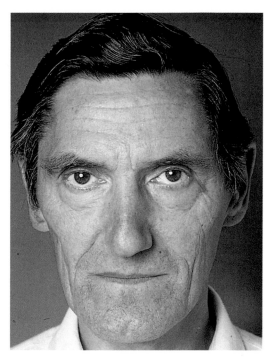

Fig. 174 (Case 11) The patient's father also exhibited marked prognathism.

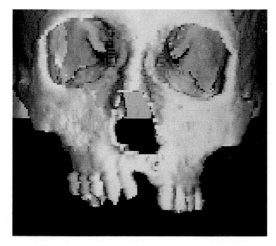

Fig. 175 (Case 11) Visualization of midfacial structures of 17-year-old patient after late secondary osteoplasty with iliac crest graft.

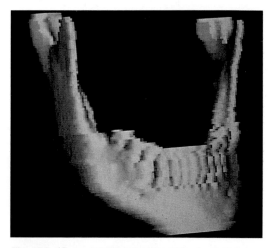

Fig. 176 (Case 11) Visualization of the lower jaw corresponding to the visualization of midfacial structures shown in Fig. 175.

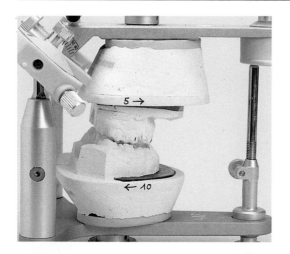

Fig. 177 (Case 11) Surgical planning using an SAM articulator. Notice the positioning alterations: 5 mm ventralization and 5 mm ventral caudalization of upper jaw, and 10 mm setback of central part of the mandible.

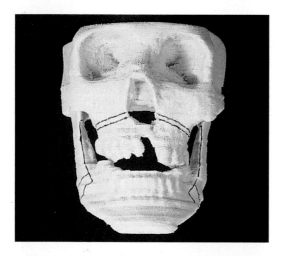

Fig. 178 (Case 11) 3-D model with osteotomy lines drawn in (frontal view).

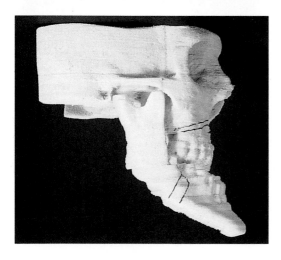

Fig. 179 (Case 11) 3-D model with osteotomy lines drawn in (right lateral view).

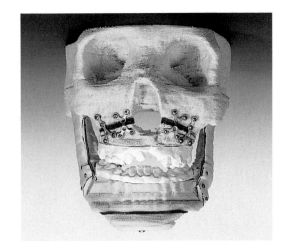

Fig. 180 (Case 11) 3-D model of surgical simulation shows osteosynthesis microplates in place (frontal view).

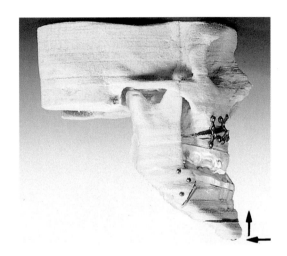

Fig. 181 (Case 11) 3-D model of surgical simulation shows osteosynthesis microplates in place (right lateral view).

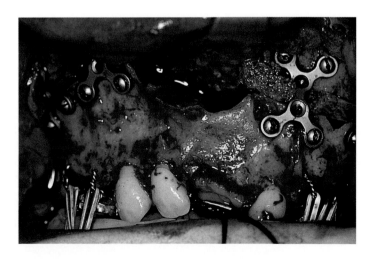

Fig. 182 (Case 11) Intraoperative situation shows preoperatively bent and resterilized osteosynthesis material; and iliac crest graft placed in position.

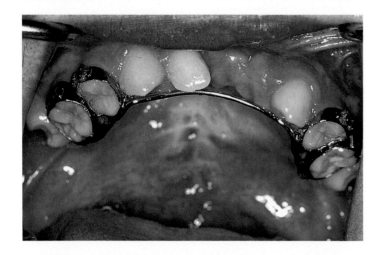

Fig. 183 (Case 11) Preoperative situation of upper dental arch.

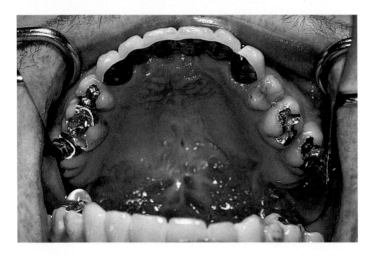

Fig. 184 (Case 11) Postoperative situation of upper dental arch.

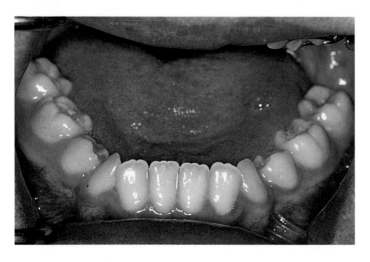

Fig. 185 (Case 11) Preoperative situation of lower dental arch.

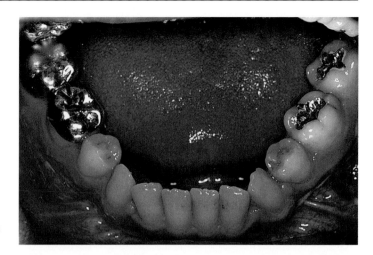

Fig. 186 (Case 11) Postoperative situation of lower dental arch.

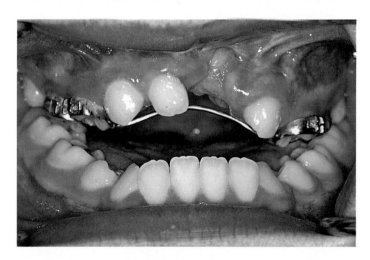

Fig. 187 (Case 11) Preoperative occlusion (frontal view).

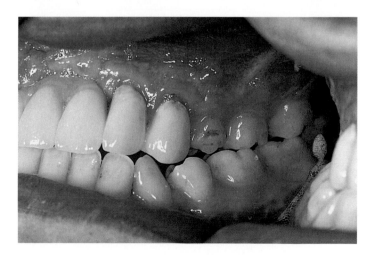

Fig. 188 (Case 11) Postoperative occlusion (left lateral view).

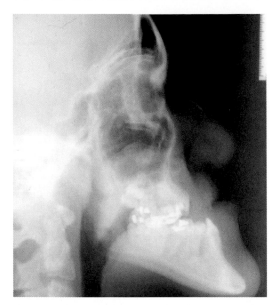

Fig. 189 (Case 11) Preoperative right lateral cephalometric radiograph.

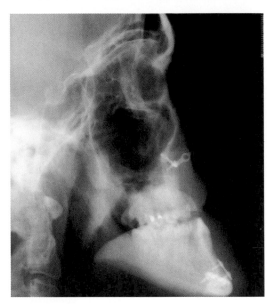

Fig. 190 (Case 11) Postoperative right lateral cephalometric radiograph. Notice the osteosynthesis material in the upper jaw after repositioning of the septum.

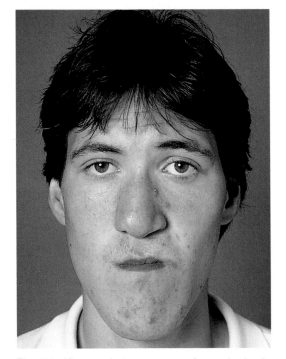

Fig. 191 (Case 11) Appearance after orthodontic treatment, before surgery.

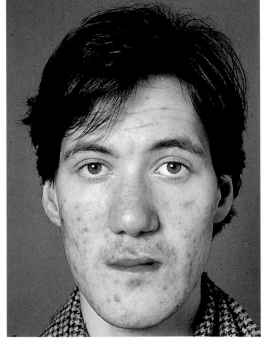

Fig. 192 (Case 11) Appearance after surgery. Other surgeries, including nose correction and genioplasty, were performed prior to the taking of this photograph.

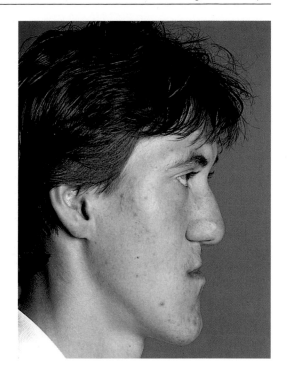

Fig. 193 (Case 11) Appearance before surgery, after orthodontic treatment (right lateral view).

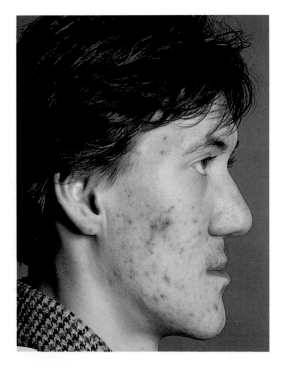

Fig. 194 (Case 11) Appearance after surgery (right lateral view). Other surgeries, including nose correction and genioplasty, were performed prior to the taking of this photograph.

Case 12 Cleft Lip and Alveolus with Severe Asymmetry
(Figs. 195 to 208)

This case, with considerable asymmetry in lateral direction, was planned as a bimaxillary surgical procedure.

The boy was born with a cleft lip and alveolus on the left side (Fig. 195). The cleft was operated on when the boy was five months old. During recall at age five signs of facial asymmetry were visible (Fig. 196).

When the present operation was planned, the patient was 24 years old. An extreme deviation of the nasal septum was visible in the CT scan (Fig. 197), and contour summation (Fig. 198) evidenced severe midline deviation.

After traditional as well as 3-D analyses (Figs. 199 and 200), the maxilla and the mandible were shifted 6 mm laterally to the right without changing the occlusion (Fig. 201). The dorsal view (Fig. 202) clearly shows the preoperative 3-D planning. Between the joint-carrying and the tooth-carrying segments of the mandible, there was a distinct gap on the left side and a close contact on the right side. Figs. 203 to 206 show pre- and postoperative radiographs for comparison. Fig. 207 shows the clinical condition prior to surgery, with a distinct asymmetrical relation between the nose and the corners of the mouth. The postoperative photograph (Fig. 208) shows the esthetic improvements achieved.

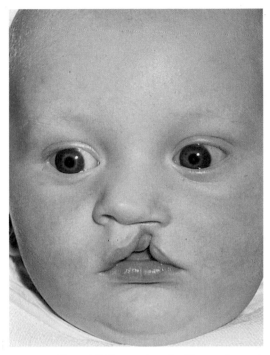

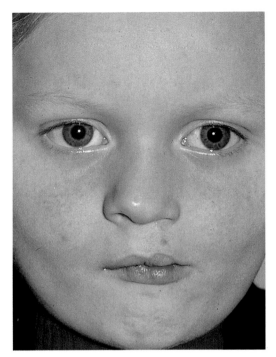

Fig. 195 (Case 12) The newborn had incomplete uni-lateral cleft lip and and alveolus.

Fig. 196 (Case 12) The patient at age five shows signs of developing facial asymmetry with midline deviation to the left.

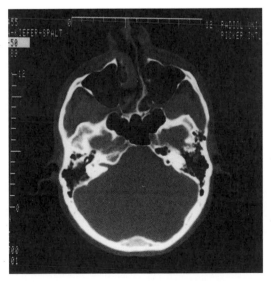

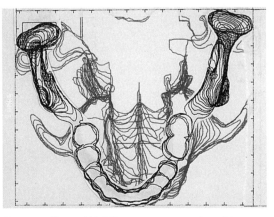

Fig. 197 (Case 12) CT scan of the adult patient, ta-ken at the level of the maxillary sinus shows deviation of nasal septum.

Fig. 198 (Case 12) 2-D contour summation of lower jaw (black) and the upper jaw (red) shows shift of the lower jaw to the left.

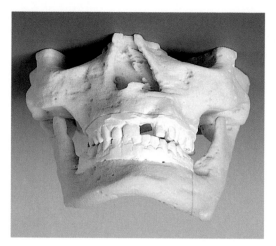

Fig. 199 (Case 12) Presurgical 3-D model (frontal view) shows midline deviation in the upper jaw.

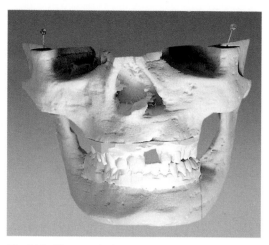

Fig. 200 (Case 12) Presurgical 3-D model (frontal view) shows deviation of both the upper and lower jaw to the left.

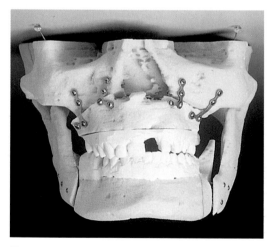

Fig. 201 (Case 12) 3-D model of surgical simulation shows movement of the mandibulomaxillary block to the right and also shows the osteosynthesis material in place.

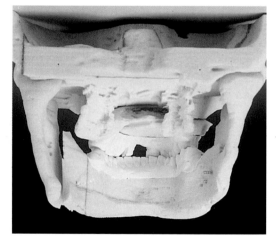

Fig. 202 (Case 12) 3-D model of surgical simulation (dorsal view) shows a large gap in the area of the sagittal split on the left side.

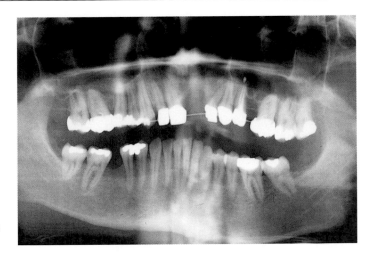

Fig. 203 (Case 12) Preoperative panoramic radiograph.

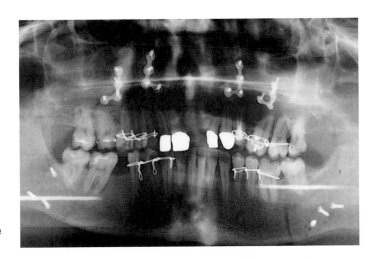

Fig. 204 (Case 12) Postoperative panoramic radiograph.

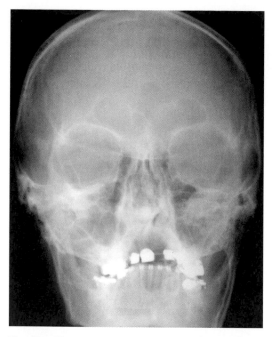

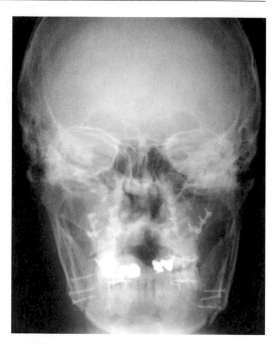

Fig. 205 (Case 12) Preoperative posterior to anterior radiograph.

Fig. 206 (Case 12) Postoperative posterior to anterior radiograph.

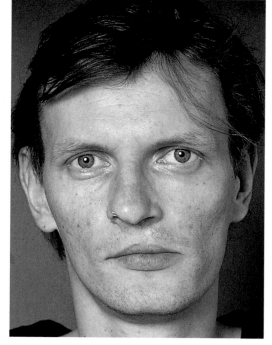

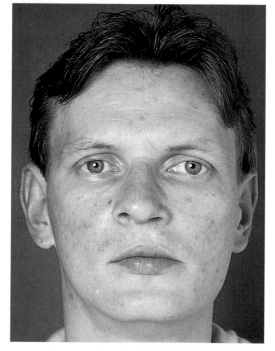

Fig. 207 (Case 12) Appearance before surgery in a case of significant facial asymmetry due to skeletal deformity (note cleft lip and alveolus on left side).

Fig. 208 (Case 12) Appearance after surgery.

Case 13 Malocclusion with Masseter Hypertrophy
(Figs. 209 to 222)

Supraclusion, or "deep bite," (Fig. 209) is not among the classical dentofacial deformities indicated for surgical intervention. This case showed elongation of the upper six-year molars after early loss of the lower ones (Figs. 210 and 211). The resulting "locked bite" combined with professional and psychological stress led to an ever decreasing ability to open the mouth. When the patient came for treatment, his mouth opening was reduced to 11 mm. Demanding expeditious treatment, he refused both orthodontic intervention and physiotherapy. The hypertrophy of the masseter muscles on both sides (Figs. 212 to 214) was correlated with a bilateral bony hyperplasia of the tuberosita masseterica (Figs. 215 and 216). Surgical therapy involved resection of the mandibular angles on both sides and bilateral resection of the processus muscularis mandibulae. After a 3-D surgical simulation (Fig. 217), the actual surgery was performed using an intraoral approach to avoid a lesion of the facial nerve and soft tissue scars.

Resections were performed by following precisely the measurements obtained from the 3-D model. Postoperative radiographs (Figs. 218 and 219) confirmed that desired results were achieved: the patient could open his mouth fully and normal mastication was ensured prosthetically (Fig. 220). The corresponding esthetic results are shown in Figs. 221 and 222.

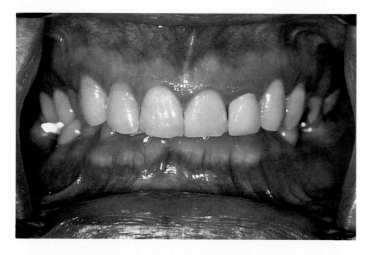

Fig. 209 (Case 13) Preoperative occlusion, supraclusion Class II (frontal view).

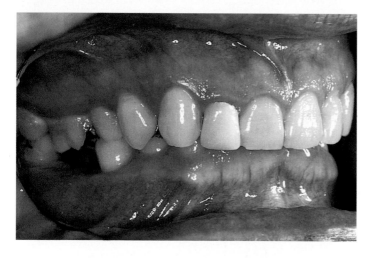

Fig. 210 (Case 13) Preoperative occlusion (right lateral view) shows an elongated first molar.

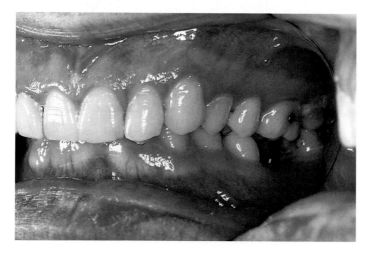

Fig. 211 (Case 13) Preoperative occlusion (left lateral view) shows an elongated first molar.

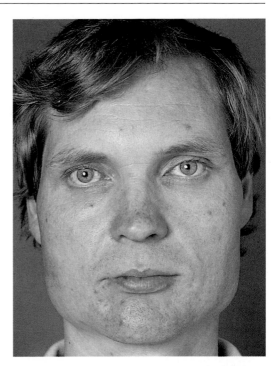

Fig. 212 (Case 13) Patient before surgery displays bilateral masseteric hypertrophy.

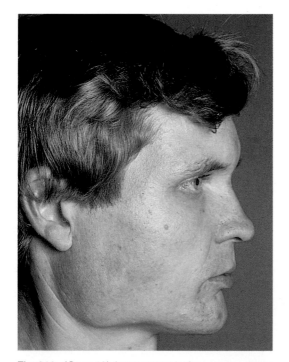

Fig. 213 (Case 13) Appearance before surgery (right lateral view), Class II masseteric hypertrophy with pronounced mentolabial fold.

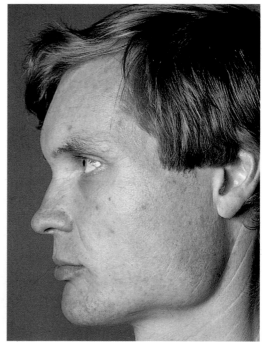

Fig. 214 (Case 13) Appearance before surgery (left lateral view), Class II masseteric hypertrophy with pronounced mentolabial fold.

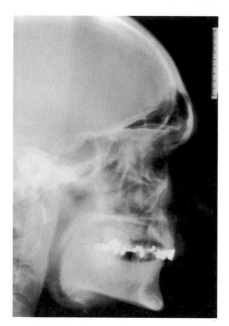

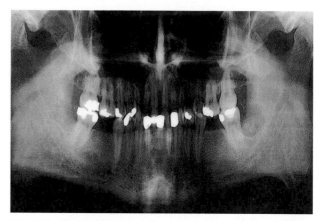

Fig. 216 (Case 13) Preoperative panoramic radiograph shows mandibular canal.

Fig. 215 (Case 13) Preoperative right lateral cephalometric radiograph shows hypertrophy of tuberositas masseterica.

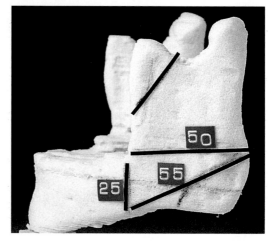

Fig. 217 (Case 13) Surgical simulation shows bilateral resection of processus coronoideus and bilateral resection of angle of mandibula.

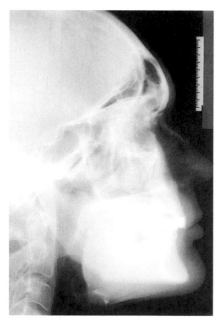

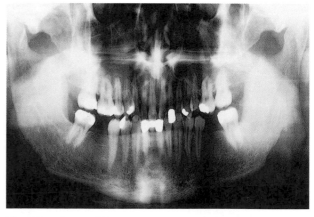

Fig. 218 (Case 13) Postoperative right lateral cephalometric radiograph.

Fig. 219 (Case 13) Postoperative panoramic radiograph.

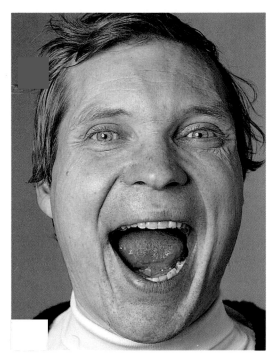

Fig. 220 (Case 13) Patient after surgery demonstrates unrestricted opening of mouth.

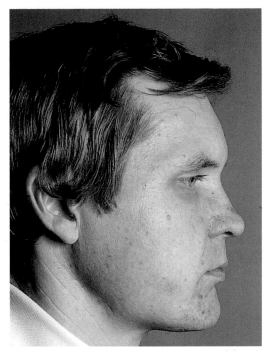

Fig. 221 (Case 13) Appearance after surgery (right lateral view).

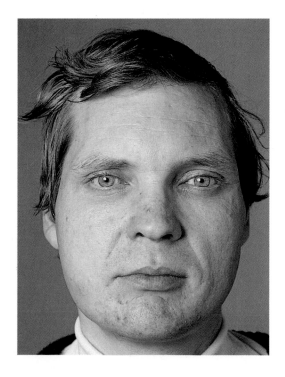

Fig. 222 (Case 13) Appearance after surgery (frontal view).

Case 14 Goldenhar Syndrome (bilateral)
(Figs. 223 to 235)

Asymmetrical deformities in the oral, maxillomandibular, and facial region offer a wide spectrum of applications for 3-D model fabrication as an aid to surgical planning.

A female patient was diagnosed with bilateral Goldenhar syndrome; 3-D technology made it possible to compare the visualization with the clinical appearance and the model with the traditional radiograph.

The bilateral expression of the syndrome led to a mandibular dysplasia and a bilateral hypoplasia (Fig. 227). The condyles showed only rudimentary development. The structure of the horizontal branches was so delicate that the model broke several times during the milling process.

The symmetrical mandibular hypoplasia produced the appearance of microgenia (Fig. 228). The finished 3-D model showed that both rudimentary condyles were firmly supported on the cranial base (Fig. 229). Due to the morphologic characteristics, surgery in the lateral mandibular region to correct the open bite (Fig. 230) was ruled out.

Instead, a maxillary osteotomy was performed in the Le Fort I plane with dorsal cranialization and closure of the open bite (Fig. 231). The hypoplasia was corrected with a two-stage plastic reconstruction of the chin, in which the fragments were held in place with three lag screws (Fig. 229).

Figs. 232 to 235 illustrate the preoperative and postoperative situations.

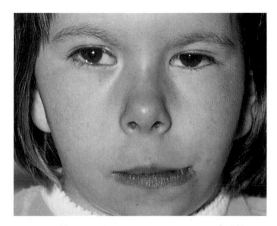

Fig. 223 (Case 14) Patient with bilateral Goldenhar syndrome (age 5).

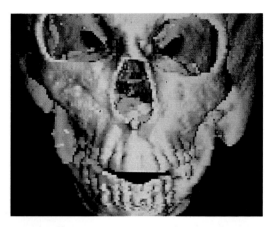

Fig. 224 (Case 14) Visualization of skull shows mandibular hypoplasia.

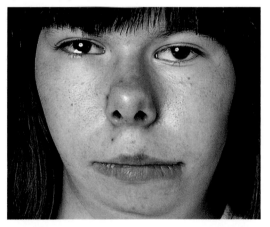

Fig. 225 (Case 14) Patient aged 18.

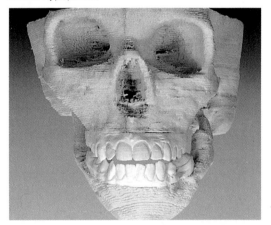

Fig. 226 (Case 14) 3-D model with plaster cast of dentition in place.

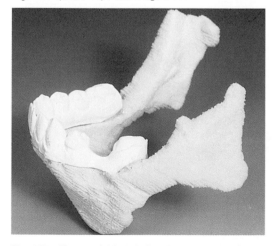

Fig. 227 (Case 14) Model of rudimentary mandible.

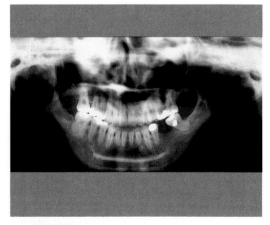

Fig. 228 (Case 14) Preoperative panoramic radiograph.

115

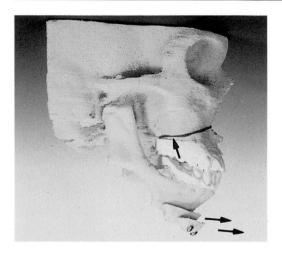

Fig. 229 (Case 14) 3-D model shows surgical simulation. Notice the dorsal cranialization on Le Fort I-level, osteotomized maxilla, and two-stage genioplasty.

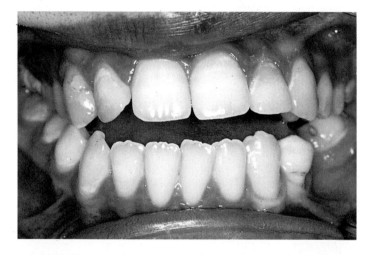

Fig. 230 (Case 14) Preoperative "open bite" occlusion.

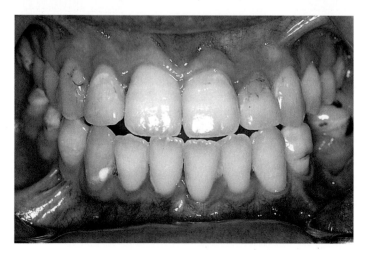

Fig. 231 (Case 14) Postoperative occlusion.

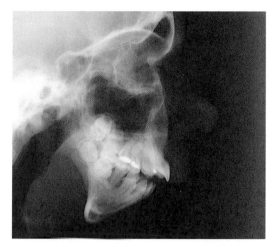

Fig. 232 (Case 14) Preoperative radiograph (right lateral view).

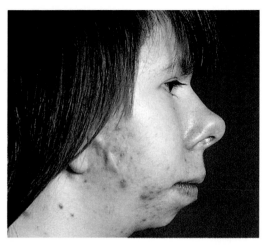

Fig. 233 (Case 14) Appearance before surgery (right lateral view).

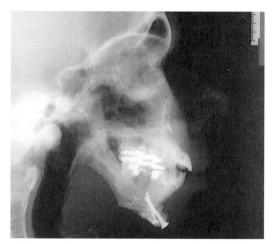

Fig. 234 (Case 14) Postoperative radiograph (right lateral view).

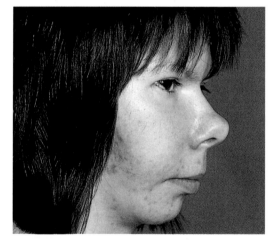

Fig. 235 (Case 14) Appearance after surgery (right lateral view).

Case 15 Goldenhar's Syndrome (unilateral)
(Figs. 236 to 250)

Unilateral Goldenhar's syndrome results in facial asymmetry, which requires skeletal therapy that must be planned differently than that for a case of bilateral expression. In 3-D model surgical simulation (Figs. 236 and 237), the maxilla osteotomized in the Le Fort I plane and the occlusal plane was made parallel to the bipupillary line. For this purpose, 6 mm of lamella was cranialized on the left in the area of the crista zygomaticoalveolaris, and on the right, 6 mm was caudalized in the area of the crista zygomaticoalveolaris. Without changing the existing occlusion, the mandible was split sagittally on the left so that the central mandibular fragment could also follow the maxilla. A severe shift toward the skull base was seen (Fig. 239), which resulted in prophylactic resection of the upper part of the left medial mandibular fragment. In the mandible on the right side, a free 5.5-cm costochondral implant was inserted to provide support on the cranial base (Fig. 238).

During the surgical procedure (Figs. 240 and 241), shifting the occlusal plane after the maxilla was fixed in its new position represented a significant step. After surgery (Fig. 242), the original preoperative occlusion was restored and the right mandible was supported by the cranial base via a rib implant. Figs. 243 to 250 show a comparison of the preoperative and the postoperative situation. The soft tissue followed the skeletal changes so the mandibular midline could be established and the lip line would run parallel to the bipupillary line.

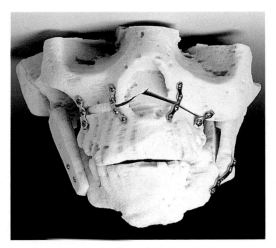

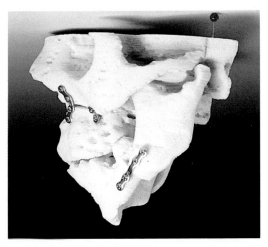

Fig. 236 (Case 15) 3-D model of surgical simulation to correct unilateral Goldenhar's syndrome (frontal view).

Fig. 237 (Case 15) 3-D model of surgical simulation (left lateral view).

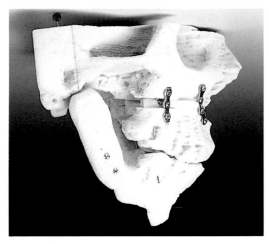

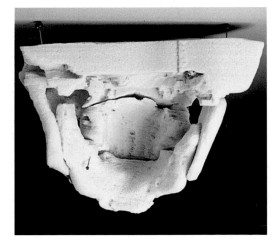

Fig. 238 (Case 15) 3-D model of surgical simulation (right lateral view).

Fig. 239 (Case 15) 3-D model (dorsal view) shows close relationship between medial mandibular fragment and skull base on the left.

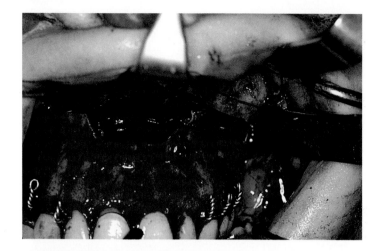

Fig. 240 (Case 15) Intraoperative situation: osteotomy of a 6-mm lamella in the Le Fort I-level (left) for moving the mandibular-maxillary block.

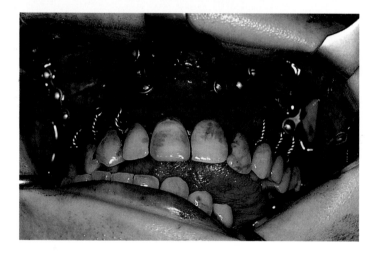

Fig. 241 (Case 15) Intraoperative situation: maxilla fixed in new position; discrepancy from original position of the mandible is clear.

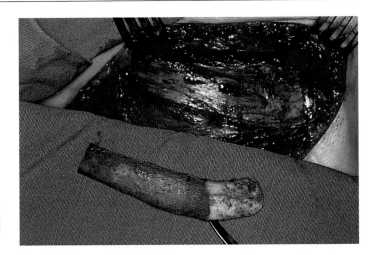

Fig. 242 (Case 15) Rib implant. The length and shape were chosen according to dimensions obtained in the 3-D surgical simulation.

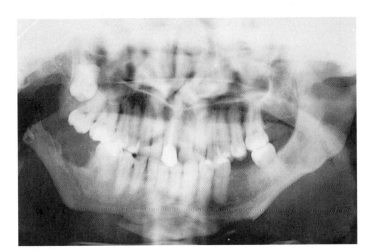

Fig. 243 (Case 15) Preoperative panoramic radiograph.

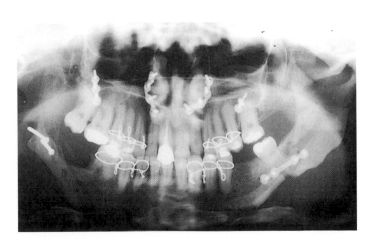

Fig. 244 (Case 15) Postoperative panoramic radiograph.

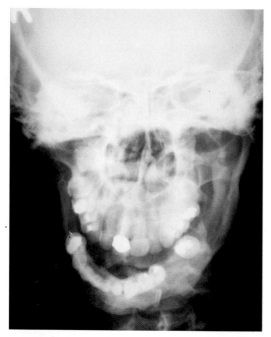

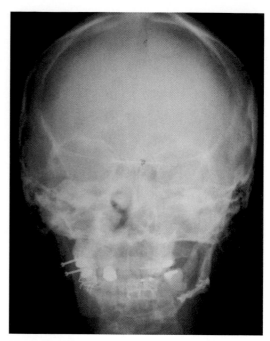

Fig. 245 (Case 15) Preoperative posterior to anterior radiograph.

Fig. 246 (Case 15) Postoperative posterior to anterior radiograph.

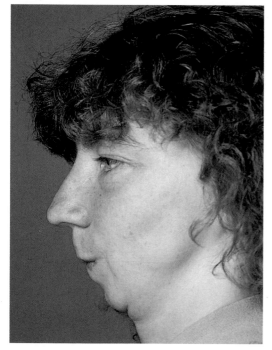

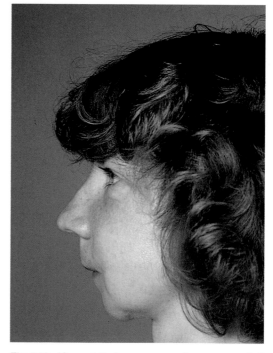

Fig. 247 (Case 15) Appearance before surgery (left lateral view).

Fig. 248 (Case 15) Appearance after surgery (left lateral view).

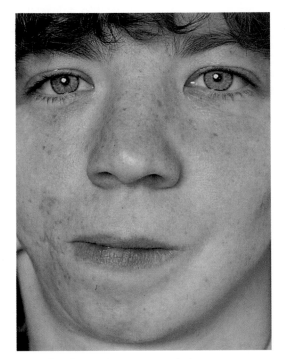

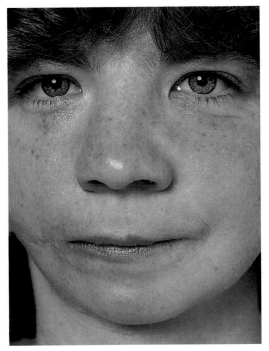

Fig. 249   (Case 15) Appearance before surgery.

Fig. 250   (Case 15) Appearance after surgery. Diagnosis: Goldenhar's syndrome, patient before surgery (left) and after surgery (right), after surgical planning with 3-D model.

Case 16 Asymmetrical Hypertelorism
(Figs. 251 to 259)

An asymmetrical hypertelorism with a lowered left orbit was diagnosed in a seven-year-old patient. This clinically obvious diagnosis was difficult to verify in either anterior or posterior orbital sections of the coronary CT scans (Figs. 251 to 253). Visualization (Fig. 254) and a 3-D model clarified the skeletal situation.

The measurements yielded by the 3-D model (Fig. 255) for surgical planning indicated that the right orbit should be shifted 5 mm in the medial direction, and that the left orbit should be shifted 5 mm in the medial and 5 mm in the cranial direction. The surgical simulation (Fig. 256) showed the expected result.

However, as unilateral orbital manipulation (Fig. 257) also produced a satisfactory result, this simpler procedure was selected. Figs. 258 and 259 show the patient before and after surgery.

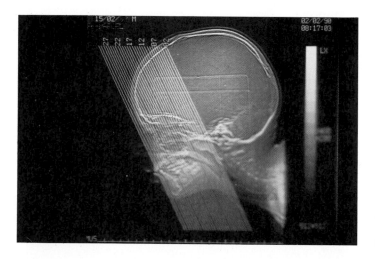

Fig. 251 (Case 16) CT scan-directed surgical planning involved a series of coronary sections of the craniofacial region.

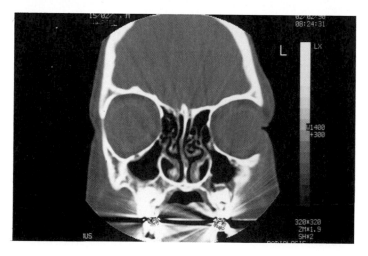

Fig. 252 (Case 16) CT scan of orbita (frontal part).

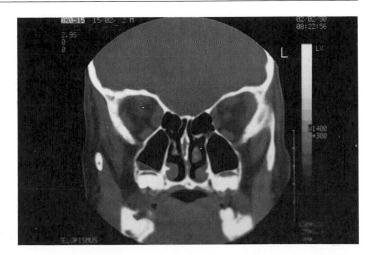

Fig. 253 (Case 16) CT scan of orbita (dorsal part)

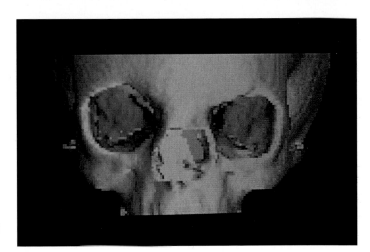

Fig. 254 (Case 16) Visualization of asymmetrical hypertelorism.

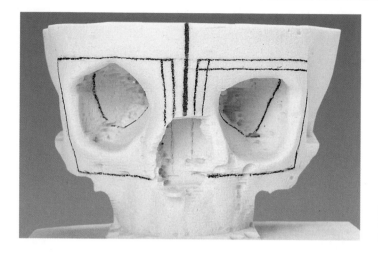

Fig. 255 (Case 16) 3-D model with lines for osteotomy for bilateral orbital movement drawn in.

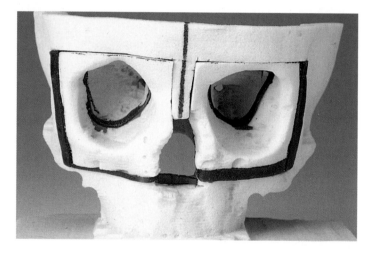

Fig. 256 (Case 16) 3-D model of surgical simulation of bilateral orbital movement.

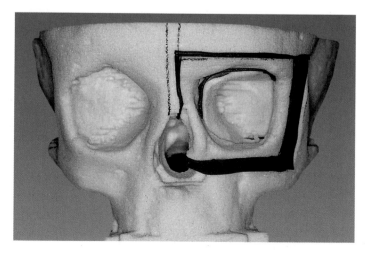

Fig. 257 (Case 16) 3-D model of surgical simulation of unilateral left orbital movement.

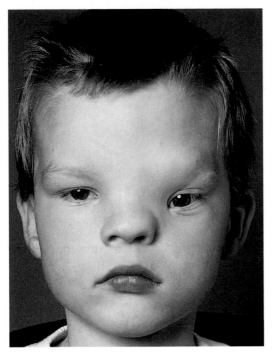

Fig. 258 (Case 16) Appearance before surgery.

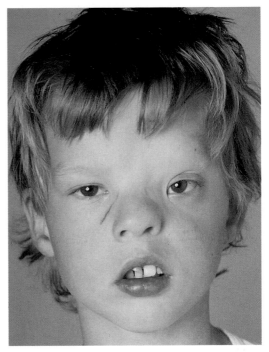

Fig. 259 (Case 16) Appearance after surgery. (Surgery performed by Prof. H. F. Sailer, M.D., D.M.D., Dept. of Maxillofacial Surgery, University Hospital, Zurich, Switzerland.)

Case 17 Partial Mandibular Resection and Reconstruction with Microvascular Pedicellate Pelvic Ridge Graft

(Figs. 260 to 270)

In a 45-year-old patient, therapy called for the surgical removal of a squamous cell carcinoma of the right oral base that was resting on the mandible. A partial resection of the bony mandible from regions 33 to 46 was performed. To prepare a model, a series of CT scans was taken. A bridge across the regions 33 to 46 was necessary for a stable model of the mandible (Fig. 260). During surgery, the preshaped resection plate could be precisely fitted to the mandible without any corrections.

Fig. 261 shows the 3-D planning of the surgical procedure involving the use of a negatively contoured support block. Through precision-fitting of the model of the mandible, the reconstruction plate could be precisely adapted to the model even after partial mandibular resection, without a change in the position of the TMJs. The resected section of the mandibular model was used for comparative measurements of the implant dimensions.

The length and insertion direction of surgical screws were determined using the

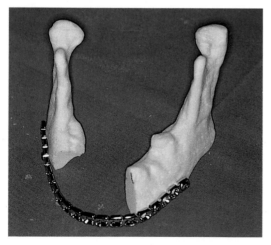

Fig. 260 (Case 17) 3-D model with adapted AO mandibular reconstruction plate.

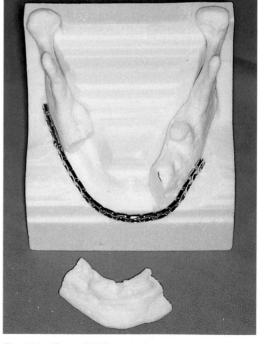

Fig. 261 (Case 17) Negatively contoured and milled support block allows for precise adaptation of the mandibular segments.

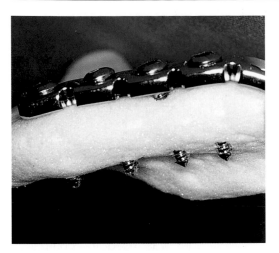

Fig. 262 (Case 17) A close-up view of adapted AO reconstruction plate shows positions of osteosynthesis screws.

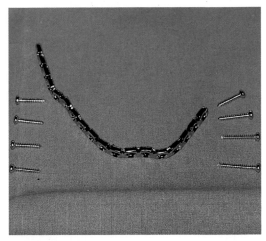

Fig. 263 (Case 17) Osteosynthesis materials for the reconstruction are prepared and ready for use after sterilization.

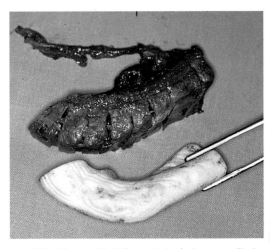

Fig. 264 (Case 17) 3-D model of the mandibular defect and pelvic ridge section is used to guide reconstruction.

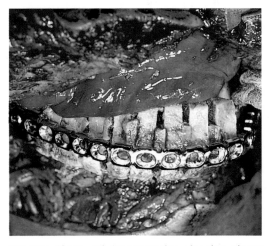

Fig. 265 (Case 17) Intraoperative situation shows fitted iliac crest graft.

model (Fig. 262). The materials needed for the osteosynthesis during the surgical procedure were sterilized and prepared (Fig. 263).

The pelvic ridge section removed for use in the reconstruction of the mandible was shaped with the help of the model (Fig. 264). During surgery, after the mandibular reconstruction plate had been positioned,

the graft was fitted into the defect to restore the bony structures of the mandible (Fig. 265). A postoperative radiograph showed symmetrical conditions in the mandibular region (Fig. 266), consistent with the clinical appearance (Fig. 267).

A panoramic radiograph taken 18 months later shows the implants that were inserted into the graft and fitted into the

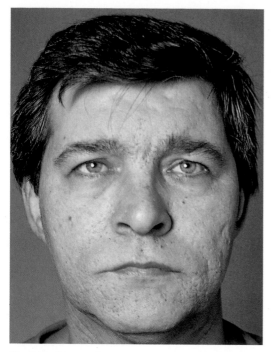

Fig. 266 (Case 17) Appearance before surgery.

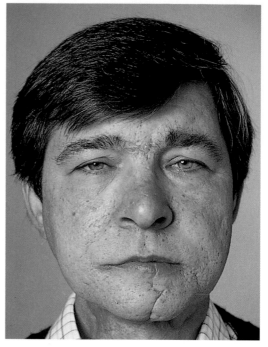

Fig. 267 (Case 17) Appearance nine months after surgery.

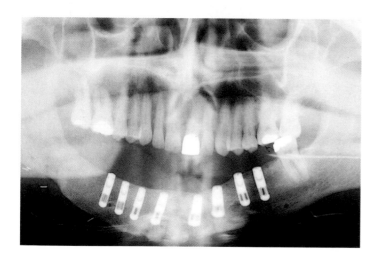

Fig. 268 (Case 17) Postoperative radiograph (18 months later) shows endosseous implants in the grafted mandibular segment.

arch of the 3-D planned mandibular implant. Fig. 268 show the postoperative radiograph and Figs. 269 and 270 the intraoral findings. To provide an intraoral cover for the defect, a jejunum graft was anastomosized microvascularly.

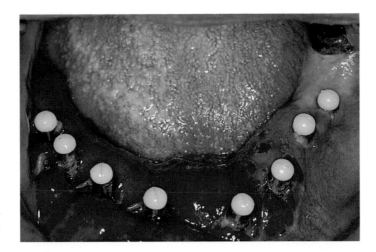

Fig. 269 (Case 17) Intraoral appearance 18 months after surgery: Jejunum graft is light red.

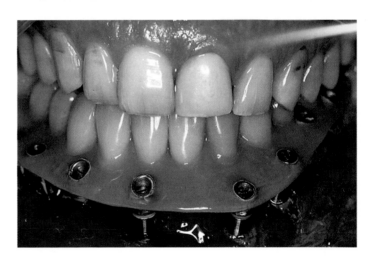

Fig. 270 (Case 17) Implant-supported prosthesis in place.

Case 18 Partial Mandibular Resection and Reconstruction with AO Reconstruction Plate and Artificial TMJ (Figs. 271 to 281)

A squamous cell carcinoma in the left mandibular area (Fig. 271) and left cheek was diagnosed in a 42-year-old patient. The mandible was partially resected, starting with region 43.

The adapted reconstruction plate (Fig. 272) was sterilized before surgery and prepared with the osteosynthesis screws (Fig. 273). By means of an individualized "key pad," screw length and positional axes could be determined on the 3-D model (Fig. 274). During surgery, each screw was placed on its previously plotted location (Fig. 275) to give ideal stability to the extended reconstruction plate. A second key pad (Fig. 276) served as a control pad to confirm the ideal position of the reconstruction plate along the mandibular margin (Fig. 277).

During the surgical procedure, the left mandibular condyle was exarticulated, and the prefabricated osteosynthesis plate was inserted (Figs. 278 and 279). The postoperative status is visible in Fig. 280 and 281. A reconstruction of the mandible with a pelvic ridge graft was planned after a year had passed without recurrence of the tumor.

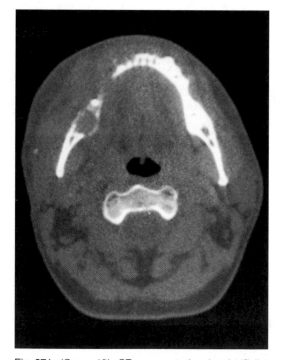

Fig. 271 (Case 18) CT scan at the level of the horizontal mandibular rami shows squamous cell carcinoma involving the left mandible and cheek.

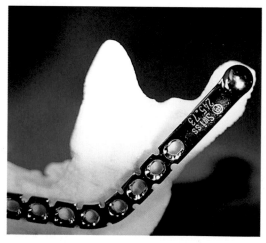

Fig. 272 (Case 18) 3-D model with reconstruction plate adapted.

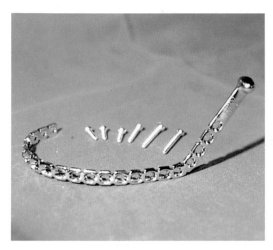

Fig. 273 (Case 18) Osteosynthesis material prepared and sterilized before surgery.

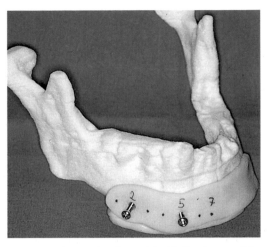

Fig. 274 (Case 18) 3-D model with first key pad for exact positioning of screw holes to optimize fixation of reconstruction plate.

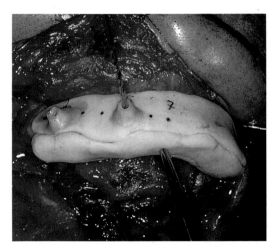

Fig. 275 (Case 18) Intraoperative situation: drilling the holes through the key pad.

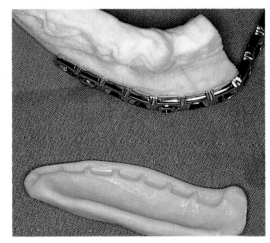

Fig. 276 (Case 18) 3-D model with second key pad for adaptation of the reconstruction plate.

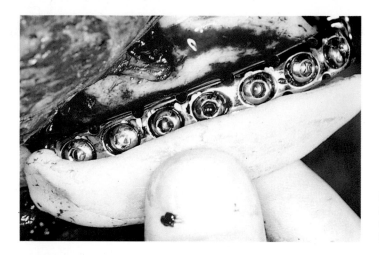

Fig. 277 (Case 18) Intraoperative situation: adapting the key pad to control exact position of the reconstruction plate.

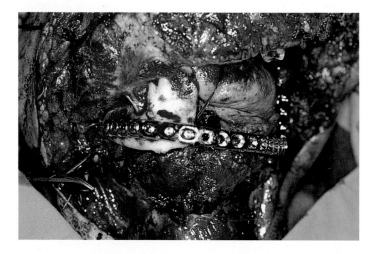

Fig. 278 (Case 18) Intraoperative situation shows osteosynthesis material in place (frontal view).

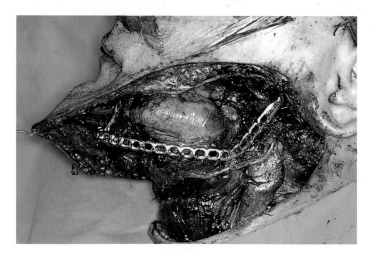

Fig. 279 (Case 18) Intraoperative situation shows osteosynthesis material in place (lateral view).

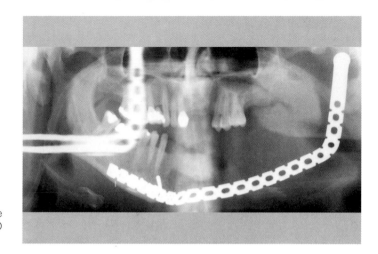

Fig. 280 (Case 18) Postoperative panoramic radiograph shows AO synthesis plate in place.

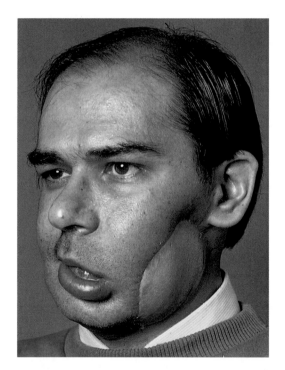

Fig. 281 (Case 18) Patient three month after surgery.

Case 19 Secondary Reconstruction Using Mirror-Image Technology

(Figs. 282 to 289)

A squamous cell carcinoma of the left tonsil and the left base of the tongue required extensive surgery in a 55-year-old patient. Specifically, a partial mandibular resection from region 33 to a point 1 cm below the left incisura semilunaris mandibular was performed, without immediate reconstruction of the bony defect (Fig. 282).

Four and a half years later, upon request of the patient, the support for the prosthesis in the left mandible was to be improved by restoring the bony portion of the alveolar process. 3-D models of the two remaining portions of the mandible, a mandibular model base, and a model of the resected segment were fabricated. The surface contours of the left fossa articularis were successfully integrated in the mandibular model base. As a model for the resected section, a mirror-image model of the mandibular bone on the right side was fabricated (so-called mirror-image technology, Fig. 283).

The model made it possible to determine the precise size and shape of the microvascular pedicellate pelvic ridge graft (Fig. 284). During surgery, the model proved to fit precisely into the existing defect, after the condyle and the processus muscularis had been resected (Fig. 285). During surgery, the microvascular pedicellate pelvic ridge graft was attached with titanium mesh to the remaining portion of the mandible (Fig. 286). A postoperative radiograph revealed symmetrical conditions (Fig. 287).

Bone scintigraphy of the skull performed after surgery revealed an accumulation of material in the area of the graft that indicated that the reconstructed mandible was satisfactorily nourished (Fig. 288). Symmetrical conditions were found after surgery (Fig. 289). The patient could be completely rehabilitated prosthetically.

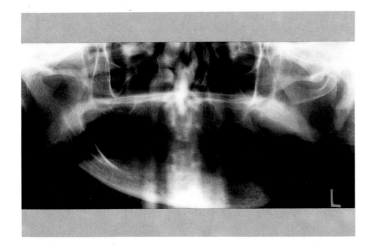

Fig. 282 (Case 19) Preoperative panoramic radiograph shows a mandibular bony defect (left) after resection of a squamous cell carcinoma.

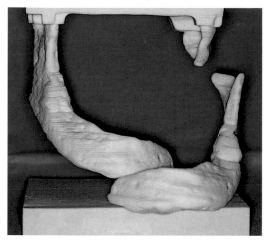

Fig. 283 (Case 19) 3-D mandibular model with mirror-image counterpart.

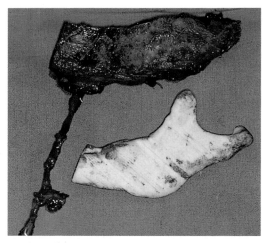

Fig. 284 (Case 19) 3-D model with microvascular pedicollate pelvic ridge graft.

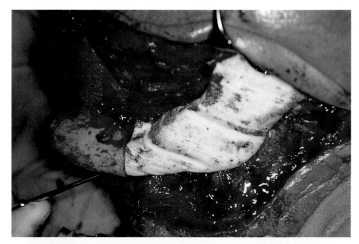

Fig. 285 (Case 19) 3-D model of graft in place to control size and shape.

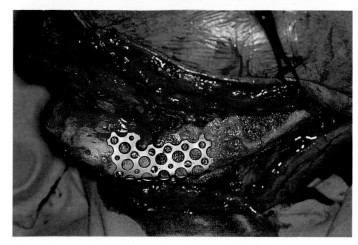

Fig. 286 (Case 19) Graft fixed with titanium mesh.

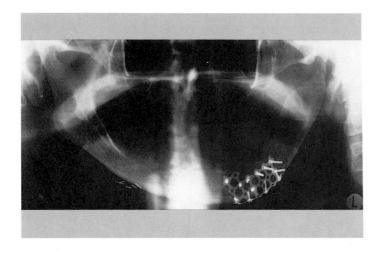

Fig. 287 (Case 19) Postoperative panoramic radiograph.

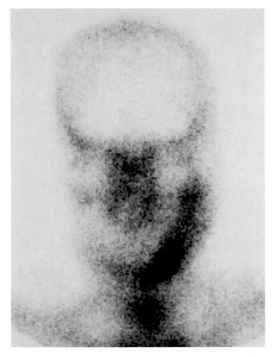

Fig. 288 (Case 19) Bone scintigram of the skull shows accumulation in the viable graft.

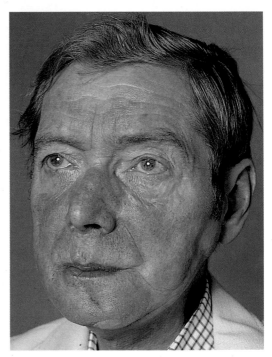

Fig. 289 (Case 19) Appearance with symmetrical structures of the lower face six months after surgery.

Bibliography

Adams L, Gilsbach JM, Krybus W, Meyer-Ebrecht D, Mösges R, Schlöndorff G. CAS – a navigation support for surgery. In: Höhne K, Fuchs H, Pizer S, eds. 3-D Imaging in Medicine. Berlin: Springer; 1990: 411–415.

Aldinger GA, Fischer A, Kurtz B. Computergestützte Herstellung individueller anatomischer Endoprothesen. Z Orthop 1984; 122: 733–736.

Aldinger GA, Weipert A. 3-D-basierte Herstellung von Hüftgelenken: Das Aldinger-System. Radiologe 1991; 31:474-480.

Andersson JE, Svartz K. CT-scanning in the pre-operative planning of osseointegrated implants in the maxilla. Int J Oral Maxillofac Surg 1988; 17: 33–35.

Arridge S, Moss JP, Linney AD, James DR. Three dimensional digitization of the face and skull. J Maxillofac Surg 1985; 13: 136–143.

Artzy E. Note: Display of three-dimensional information in computed tomography. Comp Graph Imag Proc 1979; 9: 196–198.

Baumann MA, Löst C, Radlanski RJ. 3-D-Rekonstruktion eines Zahnkeimes bei hereditärem opaleszierendem Dentin. Dtsch Z Mund Kiefer Gesichtschir 1990; 14: 477–480.

Bhatia SN, Sowray JH. A computer-aided design for orthognathic surgery.Br J Oral Maxillofac Surg 1984; 22: 237.

Brix F. Vorstellung eines Styrodurschneide- und -fräsgerätes für die Strahlentherapie. Strahlentherapie 1981; 157: 260–263.

Brix F, Hebbinghaus D, Meyer W. Verfahren und Vorrichtung für den Modellbau im Rahmen der orthopädischen und traumatologischen Operationsplanung. Röntgenpraxis 1985; 38: 290–292.

Brix F, Lambrecht JTh. Individuelle Schädelmodellherstellung auf der Grundlage computertomographischer Informationen. Fortschr Kiefer Gesichtschir 1987; 32: 74–77.

Brix F, Lambrecht JTh, Zenker W. Modellbau als neues Angebot der Radiologie für die operative Planung. In: Schneider GH, Vogler E, eds. Digitale bildgebende Verfahren – Interventionelle Verfahren – Integrierte digitale Radiologie. Berlin: Springer; 1988; 668–675.

Catone GA. Complex Maxillofacial Injuries. In: Alling C, Osbon D, eds. Maxillofacial Trauma. Philadelphia: Lea and Febiger; 1988: 419–438.

Chen SS, Herman GT, Reynolds RA, Udupa JK. Surface shading in the cuberille environment. IEEE Comp Graph Appl 1985; 5: 33–43.

Cutting C, Bookstein FL, Grayson B, Fellingham L, Mc Carthy JG.Three-dimensional computer-assisted design of craniofacial surgical procedures: optimization and interaction with cephalometric and CT-based models. Plast Reconstr Surg 1986; 77: 877–887.

DeMarino DP, Steiner E, Poster RB, et al. Three-dimensional computed tomography in maxillofacial trauma. Arch Otolaryngol Head Neck Surg 1986; 112: 146–150.

Donlon WC, Young P, Vassiliadis A. Three-dimensional computed tomography for maxillofacial surgery: report of cases. J Oral Maxillofac Surg 1988; 46: 142–147.

Düchting W. Computermodelle für Tumorwachstum. Dt Aerztebl 1988; 85: 686–689.

Dufresne CR, McCarthy JG, Cutting CB, Epstein FJ, Hoffman WY. Volumetric quantification of intracranial and ventricular volume following cranial vault remodeling: a preliminary report. Plast Reconstr Surg 1987; 79: 24–32

Ellis E III. Accuracy of model surgery: evaluation of an old technique and introduction of a new one. J Oral Maxillofac Surg 1990; 48: 1161–1167.

Engelman ED, Schnitzlein HN, Hilbelink DR, Murtagh FR, Silbiger ML. Imaging anatomy of the cranio-vertebral junction (occipito-atlanto-axial joint). Clin Anat 1989; 2: 241–252.

Ernsting M, Zeitler E, Stedtfeldt HW, Theissing J. Hochauflösende Computertomographie und ihre Rekonstruktionsmöglichkeit einschliesslich 3-D-Imaging in der Otorhinologie und der Traumatologie. In: Schneider GH, Vogler E, eds. Digitale bildgebende Verfahren – Interventionelle Verfahren – Integrierte digitale Radiologie. Berlin: Springer; 1987: 95.

Fishman EK, Ney DR, Magid D. Three-dimensional imaging: clinical applications in orthopedics. In: Höhne K, Fuchs H, Pizer S, eds. 3-D Imaging in Medicine. Berlin: Springer; 1990: 425.

Fritzemeier CU. Optische Gesichtsreliefvermessung. Fortschr Kiefer Gesichtschir 1981; 26: 1–2.

Frohberg U, and Haase L. Chirurgie simulée en modèle 3D. Rev Stomatol Chir Maxillofac, 1993; 94: 33–36.

Ghezal A, and Stucki P. 3D-Hartkopien als Alternative zur 3D-Visualisierung am Bildschirm. Informatik Forsch Entw 1992; 7: 121–125.

Giebel G, Mildenstein K, Reumann K. Fertigung von Knochenmodellen nach Computer-Tomographie-Daten zur Verwendung in Chirurgie und Orthopädie. Biomed Technik 1985; 5: 111–113.

Gillespie JE. Three-dimensional CT reformations in craniofacial pathology. Proc Br Soc Dental Maxillofac Radiol 1988; 3: 5–8.

Gillespie JE, Isherwood I. Three-dimensional anatomical images from computed tomographic scans. Br J Radiol 1986; 59: 289–292.

Gillespie JE, Quayle AA, Barker G, Isherwood I. Three-dimensional CT reformations in the assessment of congenital and traumatic cranio-facial deformities. Br J Oral Maxillofac Surg 1987; 25: 171–177.

Glenn WV, Johnston RJ, Morton PE, Dwyer SJ. Image generation and display techniques for CT scan data. Invest Radiol 1975; 10: 403–416.

Gmelin E. Bedeutung und Möglichkeiten der digitalen Bildgebung. FOCUS Med Hochsch Lübeck 1987; 4: 175–184.

Grodd W, Dannenmaier B, Petersen D, Gehrke G. Drei-dimensionale (3-D) Bildrekonstruktionen von Gesichtsschädel und Schädelbasis in der Computertomographie. Radiologe 1987; 27: 502–510.

Grüner O, Reinhard R. Ein photographisches Verfahren zur Schädelidentifizierung. Dtsch Z gerichtl Med 1959; 47: 247–256.

Guyuron B, Ross RJ. Computer-generated model surgery. J Cranio Maxillofac Surg 1989; 17: 101–104.

Haskell B, Day M, Tetz J. Computer-aided modeling in the assessment of the biomechanical determinants of diverse skeletal patterns. Am J Orthod 1986; 5: 363–382.

Helmer R, Grüner O. Vereinfachte Schädelidentifizierung nach dem Superprojektionsverfahren mit Hilfe einer Video-Anlage. Z Rechtsmed 1977; 81: 1–5.

Hemmy DC, David DJ, Herman GT. Three-dimensional reconstruction of craniofacial deformity using computed tomography. Neurosurgery 1983; 5: 534–541.

Herman GT, and Liu HK. Display of three-dimensional information in computed tomography. J Comput Assist Tomogr 1977; 1: 155–160.

Hildebolt CF, Vannier MW, Knapp RH. Validation study of skull three-dimensional computerized tomography measurements. Am J Phys Anthropol 1990; 82: 283–294.

Hing NR. The accuracy of computer generated prediction tracings. Int J Oral Maxillofac Surg 1989; 18: 148–151.

Hirschfelder H, Hirschfelder U, Beyer WF. Die dreidimensionale Oberflächenrekonstruktion knöcherner Strukturen aus computertomographischen Schnittbildern röntgenologisch schwer zugänglicher Regionen. Electromedica 1989; 57: 148–153.

Höhne KH, Bomans M, Pommert A, Riemer M, Schiers C, Tiede U, Wiebecke G. 3D visualization of tomographic volume data using the generalized voxel model. The Visual Computer 1990; 6: 28–36.

Höhne KH, Hanson WA. Interactive 3-D segmentation of MRI and CT volumes using morphological operations. J Comput Assist Tomogr 1992; 16: 285–294.

Hoffmeister B, Lambrecht JTh, Ewers R. Die dritte Dimension der Unterkieferosteosynthese. Dtsch Zahnärztl Z 1983; 38: 384.

Hoffmeister B, Lambrecht JTh. Präoperative Planung der primären Rekonstruktion bei Tumoroperationen mit mikrochirurgisch-anastomosierten Transplantaten. Wiss Ztschr Friedrich-Schiller-Univ. Jena 1990; 39: 517.

Hounsfield GN. Computerized transverse axial scanning (tomography): part I. description of system. Br J Radiol 1973; 46: 1016–1022.

Hu X, Tan KK, Levin DN, Pelizzari CA, Chen GTY. A volume-rendering technique for integrated three-dimensional display of MR and PET data. In: Höhne K, Fuchs H, Pizer S, eds. 3D Imaging in Medicine. Berlin: Springer; 1990: 379.

Hunt NP, Rudge SJ. Facial profile and orthognathic surgery. Br J Orthod 1984; 11: 126.

Imhof K. Die dreidimensionale Darstellung von CT-Bildern: Methode und Möglichkeiten. Electromedica 1989; 57: 154–159.

Jalass J. Dreidimensionale Modellrekonstruktion auf der Grundlage Magnet-Resonanztomographischer Daten. Med Diss Kiel 1992.

Kärcher H. Three-dimensional cranio-facial surgery; transfer from a three-dimensional model (endoplan) to clinical surgery; a new technique. J Cranio Maxillofac Surg 1992; 20: 125–131.

Kageyama K, Kimura K, Katakura T, Suzuki K, Aizumi J, Seino O. Helical volume CT and its clinical significance. Fukushima J Med Sci 1992; 38: 67–74.

Kanz L, Mittermayer C, Härle F. Dreidimensionale Darstellung und Differentialdiagnose von odontogenen Zysten. Dtsch Z Mund Kiefer Gesichtschir 1980; 4: 198–201.

Katagiri S, Yoshie H, Hara K, Sasaki F, Sasai K, Ito J. Application of computed tomography for diagnosis of alveolar bony defects. Oral Surg Oral Med Oral Pathol 1987; 64: 361–366.

Kawano Y. Three dimensional analysis of the face in respect of zygomatic fractures and evaluation of the surgery with the aid of moire topography. J Cranio Maxillofac Surg 1987; 15: 68–74.

Kikinis R, Jolesz FA, Gerig G, et al. 3D morphometric and morphologic information derived from clinical brain MR images. In: Höhne K, Fuchs H, Pizer S, eds. 3D Imaging in Medicine. Berlin: Springer; 1990: 441.

Kimura K, and Koga S, eds. Basic Principles and Clinical Application of Helical Scan. Tokyo: Iryokagakusha; 1993.

Kinney JH, Johnson QC, Bonse U, et al. Three-dimensional x-ray computed tomography in materials science. MRS Bulletin 1988; 13: 13–17.

Klein HM, Schneider W, Nawrath J, Gernot T, Voy ED, Krasny R. Stereolithographische Modellfertigung auf der Basis dreidimensionaler rekonstruierter CT-Schnittbildfolgen. Fortschr Röntgenstr 1992; 156: 429–432.

Kliegis UG, Schwesig W, Weigel H. An integrated system for the automatic manufacturing of organ models. Proc Nat Comp Graph Ass 1988; 3: 138–142.

Kliegis UG, Schwesig W, Weigel H, Mittelstädt R, Kortmann Th, Zenker W. Organ models for surgery planning. In: Neugebauer H/Windischbauer N, eds. Surface Topography and Body Deformity. Stuttgart: Fischer; 1990: 169–172.

Kobayashi T, Ueda K, Honma K, Sasakura H, Hanada K, Nakajima T. Three-dimensional analysis of facial morphology before and after orthognathic surgery. J Cranio Maxillofac Surg 1990; 18: 67–73.

Kreiborg S, Marsh JL, Cohen MM Jr, et al. Comparative three-dimensional analysis of CT-scans of the calvaria and cranial base in Apert and Crouzon syndromes. J Cranio Maxillofac Surg 1993; 21: 181–188.

Kreusch Th, Lambrecht JTh. Die Planung präprothetisch-chirurgischer Eingriffe mit Hilfe individueller Modellherstellung. Dtsch Z Mund Kiefer Gesichtschir 1992; 16: 44-46.

Kursunoglu S, Kaplan P, Resnick D, Sartoris DJ. Three-dimensional computed tomographic analysis of the normal temporomandibular joint. J Oral Maxillofac Surg 1986; 44: 257.

Lambrecht JTh. Dreidimensionale Versuchsanordnung zur Bestimmung von Schichtform und Schichttiefe bei Panorama-Schichtaufnahmegeräten. In: Jung T, ed.: Panorama Röntgenographie. Heidelberg: Hüthig, 1984: 33–37.

Lambrecht JTh, Brix F. Planning orthognathic surgery with three-dimensional models. Int J Adult Orthodont Orthognat Surg 1989; 4: 141–144.

Lambrecht JTh, Brix F, Zenker W. Dreidimensionale plastische individuelle Modellherstellung über computertomographische Daten. In: Pannike A, Rudolph H, eds. Entwicklung und heutiger Stand der Plastischen und Wiederherstellungsschirurgie. Rotenburg (Wümme): Sasse; 1989: 578–582.

Lambrecht JTh, Brix F. Three-dimensional operation simulation in functional skelettal surgery. J Japan Soc Cranio Maxillofac Surg 1990a; 6: 74–77.

Lambrecht JTh, Brix F. Programmazione di un intervento di chirurgia ortognatica con modelli tridimensionali. Quintessence Int 1990b; 6: 51–54.

Lambrecht JTh, Brix F. Individual skull model fabrication for craniofacial surgery. Cleft Palate J 1990c; 27: 382–386.

Lambrecht JTh, Kreusch Th. 3-D applications in oral cancer treatment. In: Fotedar ML, ed.: Oral Oncology, New Delhi: MacMillan India; 1991: 327–330.

Lang P, Genant HK, Steiger P, Stoller DW, Heuck AF. 3-D reformatting asserts clinical potential in MRI. Diagnost Imag Int 1989; 5: 32–36.

Lewin P, Trogadis JE, Stevens JK. Three-dimensional reconstructions from serial x-ray tomography of an Egyptian mummified head. Clin Anat 1990; 3: 215–218.

Lill W, Solar P, Ulm C, Matejka M. Dreidimensionale computertomographisch gestützte Modellherstellung im maxillofacialen Bereich–Ueberprüfung der Wiedergabepräzision und Anwendungsgebiete. Z Stomatol 88, 1991; 77–84.

Liu H. Two- and three-dimensional boundary detection. Comp Graph Imag Proc 1977; 6: 123–134.

Mankovich NJ, Cheeseman AM, Stoker NG. The display of three-dimensional anatomy with stereolithographic models. J Digit Imaging 1990; 3: 200–203.

Marchac D. Radical forehead remodeling for craniostenosis. Plast Reconstr Surg 1978; 6: 823–835.

Marsh JL, Vannier MW. Surface imaging from computerized tomographic scans. Surg 1983a; 94: 159–165.

Marsh JL, Vannier MW. The "third" dimension in craniofacial surgery. Plast Reconstr Surg 1983b; 71: 759–767.

Matsuno I, Kawakami M, Yamamura M, et al.. Three-dimensional morphological analysis for craniofacial deformity. J Jap Orthodontic Society 1990; 49: 291–301.

Meinzer HP, Meetz K, Scheppelmann D, Engelmann U, Baur HJ. The Heidelberg ray tracing model. IEEE Comp Graph Appl 1991; 11: 34–43.

Mildenstein K, Giebel G, Reumann K. Dreidimensionale Knochenmodelle nach Computertomographie-Daten. Fortschr Med 1985; 13: 331–334.

Mittermeyer C, Niederdellmann H. Three-dimensional reconstruction of odontogenic cysts and their relationship to teeth and bone. Path Res Pract 1979; 166: 101–108.

Mutoh Y, Ohashi Y, Uchiyama N, Terada K, Hanada K, Sasaki F. Three-dimensional analysis of condylar hyperplasia with computed tomography. J Cranio Maxillofac Surg 1991; 19: 49–55.

Niederdellmann H, Sadowy K, Reindl P. Der individuelle Unterkieferersatz nach ausgedehnten Kontinuitätsresektionen. Dtsch Z Mund Kiefer Gesichtschir 1988; 12: 330–332.

Ono I, Ohura T, Iwao F, et al. Examination of craniofacial bones associated with auricular anomaly using three-dimensional computer tomography. J Japan Plast Reconstr Surg 1989; 9: 607–621.

Ono I, Ohura T, Narumi E, et al. Three-dimensional analysis of craniofacial bones using three-dimensional computer tomography. J Cranio Maxillofac Surg 1992a; 20: 49–60.

Ono I, Gunji H, Kanek F, et al. A three-dimensional analysis of maxillofacial bones by helice volume computed tomography and its application to facial bone fractures. J Japan Plast Reconstr Surg 1992b; 9: 939–950.

Ono I, Gunji H, Kaneko F, Numazawa S, Kodama N, Yoza S. Treatment of extensive cranial bone defects using computer-designed hydroxyapatite ceramics and periosteal flap. Plast Reconstr Surg 1993; 92: 819–830.

Palser R, Jamieson R, Sutherland JB, Skiko L. Three-dimensional lithographic model building from volume data sets. Can Assoc Radiol J 1990; 41:339–341.

Pape HD, Galanski M, Rothe F. Metrischer und röntgenologischer Vergleich des Mittelgesichts nach periorbitalen Frakturen. Fortschr Kiefer Gesichtschir 1977; 22: 128–132.

Pate D, Resnick D, Andre M, et al. Perspective: three-dimensional imaging of the musculoskeletal system. AJR 1986; 147: 545–555.

Pate D, Resnick D, Sartoris DJ, Andre M. 3D CT of the spine: practical applications. Appl Radiol 1987; 5: 86–94.

Pesce Delfino V, Colonna M, Vacca E, Potente F, Introna F Jr. Computer-aided skull/face superimposition. Am J Forensic Med Pathol 1986; 7: 201–212.

Pomaska G. CAD auf dem Personal-Computer – Was darf man von 3D erwarten? CHIP Plus 1987; 5: 16–19.

Rhodes ML, Kuo YM, Rothmann SLG, Woznick C. An application of computer graphics and networks to anatomic model and prosthesis manufacturing. IEEE Comp Graph Appl 1987; 7: 12–25.

Rose EH, Norris MS, Rosen JM. Application of high-tech three-dimensional imaging and computer-generated models in complex facial reconstructions with vascularized bone grafts. Plast Reconstr Surg, 1993; 91: 252–264.

Scharffetter K, Kopf K, Mittermayer Ch. Dreidimensionale Rekonstruktion eines juvenilen ossifizierenden Fibroms. Dtsch Z Mund Kiefer Gesichtschir 1986; 10: 252.

Schellhas KP, El Deeb M, Wilkes CH, et al. Three-dimensional computed tomography in maxillofacial surgical planning. Arch Otolaryngol Head Neck Surg 1988; 114: 438–442.

Schlegel W. Computer assisted radiation therapy planning. In: Höhne K, Fuchs H, Pizer S, eds. 3D Imaging in Medicine. Berlin: Springer; 1990: 399.

Schmitz HJ, Tolxdorff Th, Jovanovic S, Honsbrok J. Einsatzmöglichkeiten der 3D-Rekonstruktion von CT-Daten. Dtsch Z Mund Kiefer Gesichtschir 1990; 14: 281–286.

Schmitz HJ, Erbe M. Ergebnisse der Biokompatibilitätsprüfung oberflächenstrukturierter Stereolithographie-Akrylharz-Implantate. Z Zahnärztl Implantol 1992; 8: 269–274.

Schwachenwald R, Müller H, Nowak G, Herb E, Borgis KJ, Arnold H. CT-gesteuerte stereotaktische Operationen zur Diagnose und Behandlung. Schleswig Holst Aerztebl 1990; 43: 51–54.

Schwarz MS, Rothman SLG, Rhodes ML, Chafetz N. Computed tomography: part I. preoperative assessment of the mandible for endosseous implant surgery. Int J Oral Maxillofac Implants 1987a; 2: 137–141.

Schwarz MS, Rothman SLG, Rhodes ML, Chafetz N. Computed tomography: part II. preoperative assessment of the mandible for endosseous implant surgery. Int J Oral Maxillofac Implants 1987b; 2: 143–148.

Seldon HL. Three-dimensional reconstruction of temporal bone from computed tomographic scans on an personal computer. Arch Otolaryngol Head Neck Surg 1991; 117: 1158–1161.

Sohn Ch, Grotepass J, Swobodnik W. Möglichkeiten der dreidimensionalen Ultraschalldarstellung. Ultraschall 1989; 6: 307–313.

Solar P, Ulm C, Lill W, et al. Precision of three-dimensional CT-assisted model production in the maxillofacial area. Eur Radiol 1992; 2: 473–477.

Speculand B, Jackson M. A halo-caliper guidance system for bi-maxillary (dual-arch) orthognathic surgery. J Maxillofac Surg 1984; 12: 167–173.

Speculand B, Butcher GW, Stephens CD. Three-dimensional measurement: the accuracy and precision of the reflex metrograph. Br J Oral Maxillofac Surg 1988a; 26: 265–275.

Speculand B, Butcher GW, Stephens CD. Three-dimensional measurement: the accuracy and precision of the reflex microscope. Br J Oral Max Fac Surg 1988b; 26: 276–283.

Steinhäuser EW, Spitzer WJ, Imhof K. Dreidimensionale computertomo-graphische Darstellung des Kopfskelettes. Fortschr Kiefer Gesichtschir 1987; 32: 97–99.

Stevens JK, Trogadis J, Parsons K, Leitao C. 3-D volume investigation: a new technologic age for the clinician and scientist. Hospimedica 1990; 8: 35–39.

Stoker NG, Mankovich NJ, Valentino D. Stereolithographic models for surgical planning: preliminary report. J Oral Maxillofac Surg 1992; 50: 466–471.

Stoll R, Stachniss V. Computerunterstützte Technologien in der Zahnheilkunde. Dtsch Zahnärztl Z 1990; 45: 314–322.

Strong AB, Lobregt S, Zonneveld FW. Applications of three-dimensional display techniques in medical imaging. J Biomed Eng 1990; 12: 233–238.

Tiede U, Hoehne KH, Bomans M, Pommert A, Riemer M, Wiebecke G. Investigation of medical 3D-rendering algorithms. IEEE Comp Graph Appl 1990; 10: 41–53.

Toth BA, Ellis DS, Stewart WB. Computer-Designed Prostheses for Orbitocranial Reconstruction. Plast Rec Surg 1988; 81: 315–322.

Udupa JK, Odhner D. Fast visualization, manipulation, and analysis of binary volumetric objects. IEEE Comp Graph Appl 1991; 11: 53–62.

Udupa JK, Hung HM, Odhner D, Goncalves R. Multidimensional data dormat specification: a generalization of the American College of Radiology-National Electric Manufacturers Association standards. J Digit Imaging 1992; 5: 26–45.

Vannier MW, Marsh JL, Warren JW. Three-dimensional CT reconstruction images for craniofacial surgical planning and evaluation. Radiology 1984; 150: 197–206.

Vannier MW. Computer applications in radiology. Curr Opin Radiol 1991; 3: 258–266.

Vannier MW, Pilgram T, Bhatia G, Brunsden B. Facial surface scanner. IEEE Comp Graph Appl 1991; 11: 72–80.

Waite PD, Matukas VJ. Zygomatic augmentation with hydroxylapatite: a preliminary report. J Oral Maxillofac Surg 1986; 44: 349.

Wallin A. Constructing isosurfaces from CT data. IEEE Comp Graph Appl 1991; 11: 28–33.

Walters H, Walters DH. Computerised planning of maxillofacial osteotomies: the program and its clinical application. Br J Oral Max Fac Surg 1986; 24: 178.

White DN. Multidimensional imaging in maxillofacial surgery. Facial Plastic Surg 1988; 5: 197–206.

Whyte AM, Hourihan MD, Earley MJ, Sugar A. Radiological assessment of hemifacial microsomia by three-dimensional computed tomography. Dentomaxillofac Radiol 1990; 19: 119–125.

Witte G, Höltje W, Tiede U, Riemer M. Die dreidimensionale Darstellung computertomographischer Untersuchungen kraniofazialer Anomalien. Fortschr Röntgenstr 1986; 144: 400–405.

Woolson ST, Dev P, Fellingham LL, Vassiliadis A. Three-dimensional imaging of bone from computerized tomography. Clin Orthop Rel Res 1986; 202: 239–248.

Yab K, Tajima S, Imai K. Clinical application of a solid three-dimensional model for orbital wall fractures. J Cranio Maxillofac Surg 1993; 21: 275–278.

Zenker W, Bielstein D, Havemann D. Neue Erkenntnisse zur Calcaneusfraktur durch den CT-Daten gesteuerten Modellbau. Unfallheilkunde 1990a; 212: 423–424.

Zenker W, Brix F, Lambrecht JTh. Dreidimensionale Weiterverarbeitung von CT-Daten zur Operationsplanung. In: Neugebauer H/Windischbauer N, eds. Surface Topography and Body Deformity. Stuttgart: Fischer; 1990b: 173–175.

Zinreich SJ, Mattox DE, Johns ME, et al. 3-D CT for cranial facial and laryngeal surgery. Laryngoscope 1988; 98: 1212–1219.

Zinreich SJ, Kennedy DW, Long DM, Carson BS, Dufresne CR. 3-D applications in neuroradiology. Hospimedica 1990; 8: 29–32.

Zonneveld FW, Lobregt S, van der Meulen JCH, Vaandrager JM. Three-dimensional imaging in craniofacial surgery. World J Surg 1989; 13: 328–342.

Zonneveld FW, van der Dussen MFN. Three-dimensional imaging and model fabrication in oral and maxillofacial surgery. Oral Maxillofac Surg Clin N Am 1992; 4: 19–33.

Manufacturer and Related Information

Software system for CT- and MRT images
(HEKplan)
Material for model fabrication:
Polyurethane foam: Ureol 5450
Polystyrene foam: Styrodur 3000S
      HEK Medizintechnik GmbH
      Postfach 1832
      D-23506 Lübeck
      Germany

Main calculator HP 9000 Series 300
Organising calculator HP Vectra
      Firma Hewlett Packard GmbH
      Hewlett Packard-Strasse
      D-61352 Bad Homburg
      Germany

Milling machine and
Integrated system for the CT-based
production of bone models: ENDOPLAN®
      MDC Medical Diagnostic
      Computing GmbH
      Zeiss Group
      Zeyestr. 16-24
      D-24106 Kiel
      Germany

Model fabrication
      Johannes Hezel, M.D., Radiologist
      ORGAMOD-3D-Modelling-
      Company
      Hasenholz 6
      D-24161 Altenholz
      Germany

Rapid Prototyping, Laser Stereolithography
and Laser Sintering by EOS GmbH
      Electro Optical Systems
      Pasinger Str. 2
      D-82152 Planegg

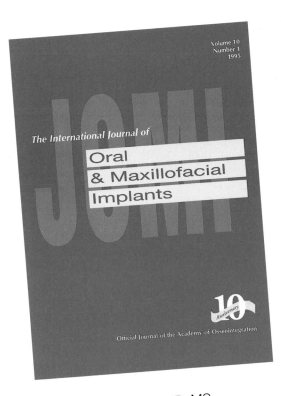

Philip Worthington/Per-Ingvar Brånemark

quintessence books

Advanced Osseointegration Surgery

Applications in the Maxillofacial Region

Advanced Osseointegration Surgery: Applications in the Maxillofacial Region presents much-awaited information on how to treat the more difficult surgical patient. The book takes readers who have prior experience in treating straight-forward implant cases and helps guide them through more demanding clinical situations.

Certain fundamental aspects are covered to provide a necessary grounding; these include the rationale of antibiotic therapy; the influence of patient age; bacteria-host interactions; radiology; and biomechanical and physiological considerations.

The clinical section of the book addresses a range of problems that often occur in practice and can tax the ingenuity of the surgeon. Such problems include severe bony atrophy; bone grafting; partially edentulous patients; and patients who have undergone ablative surgery.

Advanced, newer, and even experimental techniques are discussed (but not necessarily endorsed for general use) in the interest of helping readers to become as informed as possible on this dynamic specialty of dentistry.

Ultimately, this book builds outward from one of the author's previous works *(Tissue-Integrated Prostheses: Osseointegration in Clinical Dentistry,* Quintessence, 1985) and will be of interest to implant specialists and maxillofacial surgeons.

404 pp; 668 illus (363 in color);
ISBN 0-86715-242-7 US $ 140

To order, contact:

Quintessence Publishing Co., Ltd.
2 Blagdon Road, New Malden, Surrey KT3 4AD, GB
Tel.: (81) 8496087, Telex: 24667, Fax: (81) 3361484

Quintessence Publishing Co, Inc,
551 North Kimberly Drive, Carol Stream, IL 60188-1881
Tel.: 800-621-0387 or 708-682-3223; Fax: 708-682-3288

Quintessenz Verlags-GmbH
Ifenpfad 2 – 4, 12107 Berlin;
Postfach 42 04 52, 12064 Berlin
Tel.: (0 30) 7 40 06-0; Fax: (0 30) 7 41 50 80